FITNESS TO  DE FOR
HEALTH PROFESSIONALS

Tim Carter

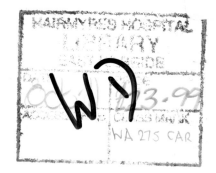

FITNESS TO DRIVE: A GUIDE FOR HEALTH PROFESSIONALS

Tim Carter

Chief Medical Adviser
Department for Transport

This publication has been endorsed by the British Medical Association and its Board of Professional Activities and Board of Science.

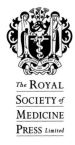

The ROYAL
SOCIETY of
MEDICINE
PRESS Limited

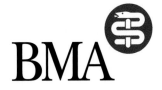

Department for
Transport

BMA

First published 2006 by the Royal Society of Medicine Press Ltd
1 Wimpole Street, London W1G 0AE, UK
Tel: +44 (0)20 7290 2921
Fax: +44 (0)20 7290 2929
Email: publishing@rsm.ac.uk
Website: www.rsmpress.co.uk

British Library Cataloguing in Publication Data
A catalogue record for this book is available from the British Library

ISBN 1-85315-651-5

Distribution in Europe and Rest of World:

Marston Book Services Ltd
PO Box 269
Abingdon
Oxon OX14 4YN, UK
Tel: +44 (0)1235 465500
Fax: +44 (0)1235 465555
Email: direct.order@marston.co.uk

Distribution in the USA and Canada:

Royal Society of Medicine Press Ltd
c/o BookMasters Inc
30 Amberwood Parkway
Ashland, OH 44805, USA
Tel: +1 800 247 6553/+1 800 266 5564
Fax: +1 419 281 6883
Email: order@bookmasters.com

Distribution in Australia and New Zealand:

Elsevier Australia
30–52 Smidmore Street
Marrikville NSW 2204, Australia
Tel: +61 2 9517 8999
Fax: +61 2 9517 2249
Email: service@elsevier.com.au

Typeset in the United Kingdom by Phoenix Photosetting, Chatham, Kent
Printed in the United Kingdom by Alden Group, Oxford

This book is printed on paper containing at least 75% recycled fibre

Reviewers

Miss Yvonne Brown
Mobility Advice and Information Service
(MAVIS), Department for Transport

Professor David Chadwick
University of Liverpool (former Chairman of the
Advisory Panel on Neurological Diseases and
Fitness to Drive)

Dr Frank Eperjesi
Department of Vision Sciences, Aston University
(member of the Advisory Panel on Vision and
Fitness to Drive)

Dr Tony Erlam
Senior Medical Inspector, Health and Safety
Executive

Dr Sally Evans
Chief Medical Adviser, Civil Aviation Authority

Professor Brian Frier*
Consultant Physician and Diabetologist, Royal
Infirmary of Edinburgh

Dr Carol Hawley
University of Warwick

Dr Peter Holden
General Practitioner, Derbyshire

Dr Tim Holt
Department of General Practice, University of
Warwick

Professor Jim Horne
Sleep Research Centre, Loughborough University

Professor Malcolm Lader*
Institute of Psychiatry

Dr Heather Major
Senior Medical Adviser, Driver and Vehicle
Licensing Agency

Mr Michael Miller*
Consultant Ophthalmic Surgeon, Moorfields Eye
Hospital

Dr Lily Read
Road Safety Division, Department for Transport

Dr Bruce Ritson*
Emeritus Consultant Psychiatrist, Edinburgh

Dr Howard Swanton*
Consultant Cardiologist, University College
London Hospitals

Professor Charles Warlow*
Department of Clinical Neurosciences, University
of Edinburgh

*Chairmen of Secretary of State for Transport's Honorary Medical Advisory Panels on Fitness to Drive.

Acknowledgements

The listed reviewers all provided expert advice on one or more chapters of this book. A range of staff in the Department for Transport and its agencies assisted with other items of information. In particular, Anil Bhagat provided statistical material, Roger Agombar advised on police and enforcement aspects, and Ela Ginalska provided support on format, style and editing.

Tom Newholm and the Driving Standards Agency prepared the colour plates.

AMA material adapted and reproduced with permission from the American Medical Association's *Physician's Guide to Assessing and Counseling Older Drivers*. Washington, DC: National Highway Transportation Safety Administration, 2003.

Hartford material reproduced with permission from The Hartford Financial Services Group, Inc., *At the Crossroads: A Guide to Alzheimer's Disease, Dementia and Driving*, © 2006 The Hartford, Hartford, CT 06115.

Regional Geriatric Assessment Program of Ottawa material reproduced with permission from *The Driving and Dementia Toolkit*, © 2001 Regional Geriatric Assessment Programme of Ottawa – Carleton.

Contents

Introduction

Almost every health professional has to advise on fitness to drive. This book aims to help you give valid advice, based on an understanding of the capabilities that a driver requires to drive safely and the effects of health-related impairments on these.

This book is primarily written as a handbook for health professionals. However, its style should also mean that it can be read and understood, possibly with the help of a medical dictionary, by other people concerned with health and fitness to drive, such as fleet managers, insurers and road safety advisers. It may also be useful to those with health problems who wish to understand the relevance of their condition to driving and how it may be assessed by health professionals and the licensing authorities.

The book is divided into five sections which discuss the following topics:

1. The capabilities required for safe driving, the effects of different forms of impairment on these, and how any risks are reduced. Responsibilities for action, in particular the role of health professionals, are described. Ways in which the personal mobility of a driver can be maintained, without compromising road safety, are outlined.

2. Sensory inputs needed for safe driving, especially vision.

3. The capabilities of mental function and of the nervous system that are needed for driving. The impairing effects of medication, alcohol and non-therapeutic drugs on driving.

4. The consequences for the control of a vehicle of limitations to the driver's movement from injury, surgery and musculoskeletal disease.

5. The main forms of sudden incapacitation that can threaten a driver's ability to remain in control of a vehicle.

Overlap between these sections is inevitable because illnesses such as stroke and diabetes can cause a range of impairments. There is cross-referencing between conditions, and to link the underlying principles of assessment to specific situations.

A driver's present state of impairment, irrespective of diagnosis, will determine current risks. Sections 2–5 discuss the use of diagnostic information. Diagnosis can be an important indicator of those manifestations of functional limitation that are less apparent and so need to be sought. Diagnosis of an individual's condition is also essential for determining their prognosis and hence the likely patterns of impairment in the future.

Because extrapolation and analogy from the – often limited – data that are available are used widely in estimating the risks of driving, it is not practicable to use a formal systematic review approach. The available evidence is summarized. Where medical conditions are being considered the chapters start with information on the risks from the common forms of impairment associated with them, followed by a discussion of the best way to assess and advise drivers.

Sound advice on fitness to drive is derived from an assessment of the driver's risk of crashing because of any health-related impairments that are likely to reduce their ability to drive safely now and in the future. The diagnosis of an individual's medical condition is just one of the factors that determines this risk. The sort of assessment that the health professional needs to make is similar to that required when determining fitness for work, fitness to travel or the scope for a return to the full activities of daily living after a major illness, rather than the normal clinical priority of diagnosing an illness in order to treat it correctly.

In the UK the Driver and Vehicle Licensing Agency (DVLA) makes many of the more complex assessments of serious illness and fitness to drive. Where this is the case this book provides information to assist you to understand the DVLA's responses to patients who are in contact with it. It does not aim to provide detailed information to enable you to take decisions on behalf of the DVLA, but it

should clarify when notification is indicated. The need to recommend that a driver notifies the DVLA is considered from the health professional's perspective rather than from that used in the DVLA *At A Glance Guide* to medical standards, which indicates the DVLA's response when a notification is received.

Many conditions do not need to be notified to the DVLA. In this situation the driver often relies on advice from a health professional. The advice needed and how you can give it most effectively are discussed for illness of short duration, after injury, following medical interventions and when medication is prescribed or purchased.

Appendix 1 provides information on a selection of tools health professionals can use to aid their assessments of fitness to drive. Appendix 2 summarizes the basis for the fitness standards used in other safety-critical tasks.

Major references on the evidence base for health-related driving risk are supplied. Sources of information and advice for health professionals and patients are also listed. The full hypertext links for those reference sources that are on the web are grouped together on the RSM Press website www.rsmpress.co.uk/bkcarter.htm to assist access.

SECTION 1: DRIVING, HEALTH AND IMPAIRMENT – MANAGING THE RISK

1. Health and the driving task

Perception, cognition and action
The road, the vehicle and the driver
Assessment of health-related impairment
Mitigation of health-related impairment and risk

Perception, cognition and action

Safe driving requires the driver to have:

- effective and reliable control of the vehicle
- the capacity to respond to the road, traffic and other external clues
- knowledge of and a willingness to follow the 'rules of the road'.

Drivers consciously learn all these skills to pass the driving test (Table 1.1) and the vast majority of people have the ability to achieve a satisfactory standard. Performance generally improves with experience and driving becomes an 'over-learned' skill that is subconsciously retained and can readily be used as required.

Impairments caused by health problems can interfere with driving performance. The task of driving can be thought of as a continuous loop, where information about the road, other drivers and the vehicle is processed by the brain, and this leads to the driver taking action to adjust the speed and direction of the vehicle and to direct their gaze to likely danger areas (Figure 1.1). The results of these actions then feed back into a further round of adjustments.

The loop is dynamic and timing is critical for making continuous adjustments in the light of new perceptions. In this respect it is not unlike the tasks of eye and movement coordination needed in sports such as football or tennis.

- Vision is the dominant sense involved.
- Visual and other perceptions convey

Table 1.1
Driving tests taken in Great Britain, 2004/5.[1]

Tests taken	1 668 000
Tests passed	706 000
Pass rate	42%
Proportion of population with driving licence	70%

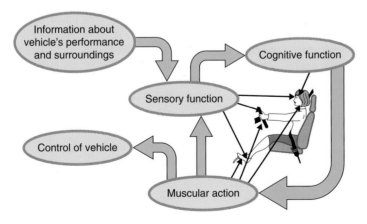

Figure 1.1
The driving task.

information such as speed, location of vehicles and other obstacles.

- The driver analyses current perceptions, based on prior training and experience about safety risks, vehicle characteristics and the anticipated behaviour of other road users.

- The intent of the journey in terms of route and destination is also used to decide the actions required, especially at junctions.

- Current perceptions, learned responses and intentions about the journey all interact, largely at a subconscious level in an experienced driver. They are converted into musculoskeletal actions so that the driver can adjust the vehicle controls using their hands and feet, and into head and eye movements to direct their gaze.

- The loop is closed by the driver observing the effects of very recent decisions about the control of the vehicle and adjusting the next ones, while also taking account of new information about the surroundings.

Any condition that impairs perception, cognition (including alertness, attitude to risk, recall) or motor function has the potential to interfere with the whole loop, and thus impair driving and make it less safe.

- This interference may be constant, as with a defect in vision.

- It may be episodic, as in a sudden loss of consciousness.

- In the longer term the time course and prognosis of the impairing condition, whether fluctuating, progressive, remitting or a mixed picture, will determine the pattern of future risk.

The road, the vehicle and the driver[2]

A wide range of external and driver variables, including health-related impairments, can influence the functioning of the loop described above and hence road safety.

Any driver in Britain shares 387 674 km of public roads with 32 million other drivers, in 26 million cars and 434 000 large goods vehicles. In addition, roads are used by other more vulnerable users such as cyclists, pedestrians – including children and the infirm – and animals.

Road

The road surface and its contours will have a big effect on car control. The driver needs to perceive changing conditions in order to respond to them appropriately. Nonvisual clues such as noise, bumps and inertial effects can be important.

Adverse weather conditions will reduce vision and, if vision is already compromised, function is especially likely to be worsened. Wet and icy roads can also reduce the vehicle's adhesion to the road surface, with the need to drive in a way that will avoid loss of adhesion and rapidly perceive the first signs of skidding.

Dark and unlit roads will pose problems if the driver has impaired visual contrast or dark adaptation is impaired, while for older drivers headlight glare is worsened by their slower adaptation to light and darkness and by increased light scatter within their eyes (Plates 1–4). Road lighting reduces these deficits. Well illuminated and clear signs help drivers respond to warnings and to direction-finding information.

Congested roads pose very different problems from empty ones. Drivers need to anticipate the behaviour of their fellow road users. Precise car control is more important. Interactions with other vehicles and their drivers are the predominant skills required.

Vehicle

Changing from one car to another reveals the differences in characteristics between vehicles – something to which most drivers rapidly adapt.

There may be very large differences, eg between cars and heavy goods vehicles or motor cycles, and such changes in vehicle require retraining to ensure safety.

In particular, the field of vision, both direct and with mirrors, can vary widely. Acceleration and braking characteristics will differ and controls may not be located in the same place. All can give rise to errors if the driver does not remain aware of the differences as they learn to respond to them.

Within the vehicle, controls for peripheral tasks such as adjusting the air temperature and flow, as well as entertainment and route-finding aids, are all becoming more complex and can distract as well as assist the driver.

The ambient conditions in the vehicle will also have an effect on the driver's performance. Overheating may encourage loss of alertness, while cold can reduce the driver's motor performance. Contaminants such as pollen or irritants can be disabling in those with allergies or hyper-reactivity of respiratory or eye mucosae.

Driver

Driver variables are the major determinant of the risk of a crash, even in the absence of any specific health-related impairment.[3] Arousal and factors that affect it, such as fatigue, alcohol and certain drugs (whether prescribed, over-the-counter or non-therapeutic) all influence a driver's performance.

Mood and interactions with passengers, children in the back, other drivers or those at the other end of a conversation on even a hands-free mobile phone, have not only an effect on mood but also serve to divide attention between safe driving and another task, creating executive and memory conflicts over priorities.[4]

Experience will lead to repertoires of safe behaviour but also to short cuts in driving behaviour that can increase risk. A young driver who has recently passed their test may be able to meet the test requirements but their driving behaviour, especially with their own peer group, can lead to unsafe actions and a high crash rate. By contrast many drivers with a long-term record of safe driving have developed their own patterns of driving behaviour. These may not be fully in accord with the requirements as examined in the driving test, and this has implications for the assessment of driving performance later in life. When this is done the assessor has to develop an opinion of the driver's overall safety rather than of strict compliance with driving test requirements.

With advancing age uncorrected visual function is restricted to a limited range of distances and many responses become slower; as a consequence drivers may adopt a cautious approach that leads to changes in driving performance that can irritate other road users. The increased crash risk in older drivers is not great and they contribute to relatively few casualties in other road users. However, the increased frequency of health problems and medication use with age will have implications for the performance of some older drivers.

Assessment of health-related impairment

The options for assessing health-related impairment depend on the time course and stability of the condition underlying it.

- *Fixed impairments* such as visual defects or amputations can be assessed in an individual. The actions required will be determined by whether the impairment, as found in that individual, is likely to interfere to a significant degree with the loop of perception, cognition and action on which safe driving depends (Figure1.1).

- Conditions where there is a *risk of sudden incapacity*, such as epilepsy, cardiac arrhythmias or hypoglycaemia, can only be assessed in terms of the probability of a recurrence while driving. For this, actuarial data based on the prognosis of others with a similar condition need to be used. The assessor can make a more precise estimate of individual risk if it is possible to stratify risk among those with a particular condition, eg the severity of a head injury and the subsequent probability of a seizure.

- Many health problems create a relatively *short period of impairment*, eg hay fever, an accident or surgery, or the effect of the one-off use of an impairing medication. Again, advice has to be based on the performance of other people with a similar condition but may be tempered by the driver's own perceptions, eg of problems with pedal control because of pain after a foot injury. Because of the timescale, the main means of reducing risk is often the good sense of the driver, aided by a health professional's advice, eg about the effects of a medication on alertness.

- Some conditions may lead to *fluctuating impairment over a long period*, eg in fatigue and level of muscle control associated with multiple sclerosis. More problematically, a continuing drug or alcohol habit is likely to cause dose-related impairment. Sanctions may be needed where the driver lacks self-awareness about the impairment or where risky behavioural traits underlie the condition. However, where the driver has good recognition of fluctuations, they can validly take decisions on driving, provided there is a pattern of activity that allows driving to be stopped when impairment increases. Regular oversight by a health professional and sometimes the DVLA is likely to be needed to take stock of the pattern of fluctuations and to identify any progressive impairment.

- *Progression of a condition* such as a dementia or motor neurone disease may indicate that the driver's capacity to drive safely should be assessed relatively frequently. At the same time the driver and their carers need to be encouraged to plan ahead so that when it is no longer safe for them to drive they can stop with as many of their mobility needs as possible resolved. Where, as in dementia, insight is lacking this may be difficult to achieve.

Mitigation of health-related impairment and risk

Risk reduction may be achieved by a range of methods:

- self-regulation of driving so as to take account of any perceived impairments
- advice to restrict driving, eg at night if there is a glare problem
- treatment of the impairing condition
- provision of a remedy such as distant-vision glasses
- use of less impairing remedies such as the relatively non-sedating antihistamines
- choice of a vehicle to accommodate any limitations in function, eg good all-round vision and mirrors
- vehicle adaptation with modified controls, eg to enable the driver to operate all controls by hand if there are limitations on leg and foot movement
- issue of a licence that limits the pattern of driving, eg to a limited distance from home or to daylight hours only (not currently used in the UK)
- frequent review, with re-licensing only if the impairment has not progressed
- cessation of driving, based on personal decision, advice or withdrawal of licence.

The nature of the condition itself may also be important in that the driver may be able to take mitigating action. Thus, while incapacity in a seizure can be instant, the majority of acute cardiac events have a short warning period before there is incapacitating cerebral anoxia. This often enables the driver to pull off the road. Hypoglycaemia in insulin-using diabetics can often be avoided by good personal management or by taking glucose when early symptoms arise.

Summary

- Safe driving requires the integration of perception, cognition and motor function. Impairments of all sorts, including those associated with ill-health, can interfere with this.

- Health-related impairments are only one contributor to reduced driving performance and are only responsible for a fraction of the total risk.

- The nature of the driving task and the features of any impairing health condition influence the way in which the risks of conditions need to be assessed, and the advice to be given.

- Health professionals have a key role in mitigating health-related impairment and thus reducing the risk of a crash, while enabling as many people as possible to stay safely mobile.

References

1. Department for Transport. *Transport Statistics of Great Britain 2005*. London: HMSO: 167 (with additional material from the Driving Standards Agency). www.dft.gov.uk/stellent/groups/dft_transstats/documents/divisionhomepage/038093.hcsp

2. Evans L. *Traffic Safety*. Bloomfield Hills, Ml: Science Serving Society, 2004. www.scienceservingsociety.com

3. Evans L. *Traffic Safety and the Driver*. New York: Van Nostrand Reinhold, 1991.

4. Stutts J, Feaganes J, Reinfurt D, *et al*. Driver's exposure to distractions in their natural driving environment. *Accid Anal Prev* 2005; **37**: 1093–1101.

2. Driver impairment and the risk of a road crash

Road, vehicle and driver factors in crashes

Investigating the risks from health-related impairment

Other causes of impairment leading to crashes

Consequences of a dangerous incident

Road crashes cause injury or death to the driver, passengers and other road users, vehicle and property damage, and congestion and delay.

Probability of a dangerous incident

The probability of a dangerous incident will be inherently related to time at the wheel or distance driven.

Driver impairment may contribute to a crash. However, the risk from some forms of impairment may depend, at least in part, on driving conditions, such as poor visibility for those with limitations to vision; complex decision-taking on fast busy roads for those with cognitive impairment; or tedious driving on empty roads for those with sleep disorders.

For a *suddenly incapacitating event*, linking the time of the event to a dangerous incident is straightforward. Where there is a level of *continuing impairment*, risk will depend on the likelihood of sensory clues being missed, cognitive analysis being flawed or car control being inadequate.

All the above risk factors will be related in quite complex ways to the normal clinical indicators of disease or to any functional limitations.

Consequences of a dangerous incident

The consequences of a dangerous incident will mainly be determined by factors such as the type of vehicle driven and the road conditions.

Impairment plays only a small part in terms of ability to mitigate secondary damage. Frailty of driver or passengers, as in the elderly, may increase severity of harm.

In crowded areas where there are large numbers of vulnerable road users, such as pedestrians or cyclists, serious injury is more likely.

Road, vehicle and driver factors in crashes

Estimates of the relative contributions of road conditions, vehicle and driver to crashes have been made (Figure 2.1):[1-4]

- About one-third have multiple causes.
- In around two-thirds a road user, most commonly a driver, is the major cause.
- However <5% are solely attributable to the vehicle and/or road condition.
- Hence >95% are substantially attributable to the driver or another road user.

Most evidence suggests that, in the framework of current driver licensing, advice, and personal decision-taking, impairments that are directly health related are only small contributors to overall accident risk.[5] However, forms of impairment such as sleepiness and alcohol, drug and medication use, where health problems may underlie the impairment, are major contributors.

Investigating the risks from health-related impairment

It is not easy to study the role of health as a cause of impairment leading to crashes and dangerous incidents on the road. One important consideration is the correct denominator, or measurement of the size of the at-risk group, in calculating any ratios. The ratio normally used to calculate the risk rate in road statistics is the number of accidents per unit of distance

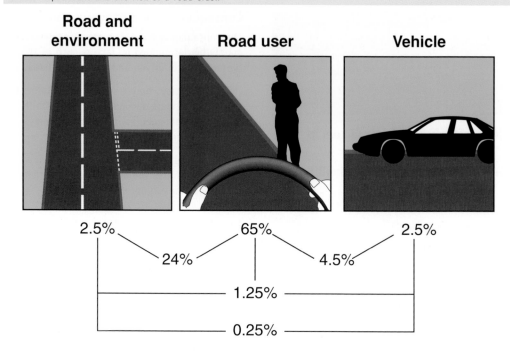

Road and environment   **Road user**   **Vehicle**

2.5%   65%   2.5%

24%   4.5%

1.25%

0.25%

Figure 2.1
Percentage of crashes attributable to road conditions, road users, vehicles alone (top line) and in combination (lower lines).[1]

driven (eg fatalities per million kilometres driven). However, for some medical conditions, especially those causing sudden incapacity, the appropriate ratio will be the number of crashes or acute episodes of incapacity per number of hours at the wheel (eg predicted rate of seizures per year – with estimates of time at the wheel for different groups of drivers). This may not correlate well with rates based on the distance driven, as high-risk groups may well drive more slowly and restrict themselves to making short journeys on local roads.

Estimates of crash risk in drivers with impairment from health problems can be made using several usually less than perfect sources of data.

- *Police accident investigations* are primarily made for enforcement purposes and do not reliably record medical factors. They may provide some incidental indications

of acute incapacitating conditions and of the extent of non-declaration of health problems to the licensing authorities. Special studies may be set up where the police collect additional information or where additional investigators work with the police at the scene of an accident (Table 2.1). Some other countries do estimate medical impairment as a routine part of police practice.

- *Crash data on groups with specific health conditions* do not usually show any major difference in risk from the rest of the driving population. Such studies will only include those who have declared their condition and been allowed to drive, and hence are assumed to be at low risk, and those who have failed to notify the licensing authority, a group who are unlikely to give correct answers about health in any investigation of a crash. In

Table 2.1
Contributory factors to accidents, Great Britain, 2000–2004, as percentages.[4]

Impairment	Fatal	Serious	Slight	Total
Alcohol	14	11	6	7
Illness	4	2	1	1
Fatigue	4	2	1	1
Drugs	3	1	1	1
Disability	1	1	0	0
Distraction–stress/ state of mind	4	2	2	2

Note: Estimates are based on sample survey of police who collected additional data when investigating vehicle crashes.

addition, drivers with impairments often modify their driving habits, eg by avoiding night driving if their vision is poor. Correction for age and for differences in the pattern of driving because of the condition can be complex. Behavioural traits linked to the condition, such as a reluctance in those with depression to initiate actions including travel, may also skew results.

- *Crash and citation (police warning and enforcement action) records* in driving licence holders with declared medical conditions can be compared with the rest of the licence holders in the same jurisdiction. Several US states, such as Utah[6] (see p. 12) have undertaken such studies, which provide information on relative risk for those with common conditions but are usually unable to identify the causative factors in the subsequent incidents. These studies have generally found a higher but not marked increase in risk in a range of conditions, some of which are also associated with frailty and impaired cognition and are more common at advanced age.

- *Population-based studies of road accidents.* The rarity of accidents in any one driver (all reported accidents 34.1, accidents resulting in death or serious injury 4.0, fatal 0.4 – all rates expressed per million vehicle kilometres) means that very large populations would be needed to study the causation of accidents.[7] Detailed investigation at the accident site and of the driver immediately after the event and linkage with prior medical history would be needed to assess whether health-related impairment played a part in causation. Given other evidence on the rarity of health-related impairment as a contributor to accidents, the power of a study with less than the national population of drivers involved would be low. Such investigations have not been undertaken.

- *Driving simulator studies* allow the effects of impairment to be studied without a risk of crashes (Figure 2.2). This approach is unsuitable for episodic forms of impairment, but can be used to identify and analyse the risks to safe driving from stable defects such as limitations on vision. Driving simulation has been used to study the transient impairments caused by alcohol, drugs – both recreational and prescribed – and fatigue. There are problems with extrapolation, and even the most sophisticated simulators do not contain all the cues present in a real car. This can mean that drivers with less than full cognitive function find the shift of reality needed to drive in a simulator very difficult and hence their performance will be worse than in a real vehicle.

- *Driving on public or private roads with*

experimental impairment has been used occasionally to study driving performance. Studies have used both simulated and real impairment, eg by creating visual acuity or field limitations using lenses or by the controlled administration of alcohol or cannabis. The subject's competence to drive is then assessed on either public or private roads, using dual-control cars, but there are practical and ethical limitations to this approach because of the risk of a crash.

- *Studies unrelated to driving* can be used to extrapolate risk, especially the relative risk for different sub-groups with the same health condition. This has been applied in particular to conditions causing sudden incapacity, such as seizure, cardiac event and hypoglycaemia from insulin. The results

of clinical epidemiology studies can be used to predict future event rates and these are used to postulate whether a driver has a high risk of incapacity at the wheel. There are some limitations to the use of such data. Any completed study will represent the pattern of risk, diagnosis or clinical intervention at the time when it was done. It will relate to the population studied, which may differ from the UK driving population. In areas such as cardiology, where new biochemical parameters, such as troponin level for the diagnosis of myocardial infarction, have come into use, the definition of the condition of concern may shift. Where new approaches to keeping blood vessels patent, such as stenting, become the norm, recurrence data based on other forms of angioplasty may no longer be relevant.

The Utah study[6]

Utah has a driver licensing system based on driver self-reporting of impairing medical conditions, but differs from the UK in issuing licences restricted, for example, by time of day, area, etc. This study used state-wide record linkage to determine the crash and citation rates for all drivers who reported 12 common types of medical condition, distinguishing between those with and without restrictions. Their rates were compared with those of age-matched controls with the aim of correcting for variations in driving pattern associated with work and leisure activities.

- 55 000 drivers with medical conditions were included in the study. Of these 51 000 had unrestricted licences.

- Citation rates for the medical condition group as a whole were only marginally elevated.

- Total crash rates were elevated by around 30% in the group with medical conditions.

- At-fault crash rates were elevated by around 50% in the group with medical conditions.

- For citations there were significant increases in crash rates amongst those with learning/memory, psychiatric and drug and alcohol problems, as

well as in drivers with reduced visual acuity or with functional limitations on motor performance. Only for drugs, alcohol and visual acuity were these increases found in both restricted and unrestricted drivers.

- The relative risk of a crash was increased for several conditions, with a higher relative risk when just the police reports which identified that the driver was at fault were analysed. Increases were shown for: diabetes, pulmonary disease, neurological conditions, epilepsy, learning/memory disorders, psychiatric conditions, drug and alcohol users, visual acuity and musculoskeletal disorders.

- The authors recognize the limitations of such a study based on self-reports which does not control in more detail for patterns of driving and, in particular, takes no account of the extent to which different groups of drivers self-police their driving to avoid patterns of car use that are subjectively difficult for them.

The results from this study are being used in a number of countries as the basis for setting priorities for reducing the risk from health-related impairment in drivers.

Data on prognosis and risk will always lag behind new and changing forms of therapy. The concern in relation to fitness to drive, eg in heart disease, is about the probability of relatively short periods of incapacity with sudden onset. Many of the studies used to make such estimates were primarily designed to measure recurrences of disease using the incidence of consultation, hospital admission or death as markers. Extrapolation based on the recurrence rates of these markers in different sub-groups assumes these recurrence rates correlate with the incidence of sudden incapacity.

Thus the quality of the evidence on road safety risks from various types of health-related impairment is variable. It is dependent on assumptions and extrapolations that have to be made in order to estimate risk while driving. It has to be used with caution, and supplemented with advice from those with relevant expertise, when developing standards or when taking decisions about or advising on fitness to drive.

Results from such approaches form the basis for the condition-specific advice outlined in later chapters. A small number of major reviews draw together most of the available information on risk.[8–10]

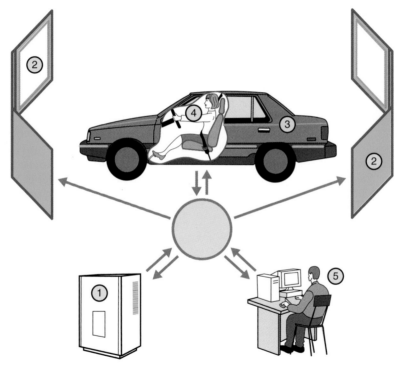

1 Computer programmed to produce images of road layout and traffic.
2 Front and rear screens for projection images. Image adjusted in response to use of car controls.
3 Stationary car with normal driving position, controls with correct feel. Engine and road noise simulated. Inertial effects of acceleration, braking, turning mimicked.
4 Driver under test: normal, real or simulated impairment.
5 Recording and analysis of driver performance: speed, road position, use of controls, response to risks. Physiology, eye/head movements and subjective state may be recorded.

Figure 2.2
Diagram of components of a driving simulator.

Other causes of impairment leading to crashes

Alcohol, medication, drugs and fatigue

The evidence base on impairment from alcohol is well defined using crash risk data (Table 2.2). It shows an increase that can be correlated with intake and with breath and blood alcohol levels.[12] Most alcohol risk is dealt with by the police and the courts. By contrast the role of health professionals (apart from as educators and dealing with the consequences of acute intoxication) is usually focused on dealing with dependency, which carries a high risk of recurrent incidents (see Chapter 14).

Simulator studies have provided evidence on the impairing effects on driving of therapeutic medications and recreational drugs. Such studies have also shown how medication and non-therapeutic drugs often interact synergistically with alcohol. Evidence about the risk of crashes is much more limited for medications and drugs than for alcohol, and it is only available for a few of the most widely used compounds. Those who have died in road crashes have been investigated for the presence of common medications and drugs as well as levels of alcohol (see Chapter 14).

There is good evidence that fatigue and sleep at the wheel are important causes of crashes. The pattern of crashes and casualties indicates that most of the risk is not related to medically identified sleep disorders but to sleep deprivation in otherwise fit people, largely young males.[13] The correlation between sleep deprivation and the exacerbating effects of even small quantities of alcohol has been studied using simulators. However, sleep disorders do contribute to this risk and sufferers have a high relative risk of crashes. Such disorders can often be remedied, leading to reductions in crash risk as well as improvements in general well-being. These are discussed separately in Chapter 21.

Age and crash risk

There are good data relating the age of drivers to crash risk. All measures of risk, whether casualties or insurance claims, identify young drivers, especially males, as the highest risk group. However, now that most drivers obtain their licence in their late teens or early 20s it is not possible to separate out the effects of young age from those of inexperience (see p. 41).

Driver behaviour

Many of the common antecedents to a crash, such as speed and risk taking, reflect behaviour traits in the driver or drivers involved. There is good evidence that some personality traits and cognitive styles are important determinants of crash risk.[14,15] However, such traits do not generally come within the ambit of the health professional except where they form part of a severe personality disorder or when expressed as, for example, alcohol or drug dependence. There are no measurable features of behaviour (other than a record of previous poor driving that has led to conviction) and which are sufficiently validated to be of statutory use as a basis of selection for or exclusion from driving. A driver's behaviour may change as a consequence of a head injury and in neurological conditions such as stroke or multiple sclerosis. Medication, especially when used to treat mental ill-health, may help to improve adverse behavioural features. However, some medication-induced conditions, such as hypoglycaemia from insulin, can sometimes cause drivers to become disinhibited and to take risks.

Table 2.2

Road crashes attributed to alcohol in Great Britain, 2003.[11]

Deaths	580 (17% of total fatal crashes)
Serious injury	2530
Slight injury	15 820
All	18 990 (7% of total crashes)

Consequences of a dangerous incident

There are significant differences in the consequences of a dangerous incident for different types of vehicle and user.[16]

For all forms of impairment, self-regulation or adaptation of driving pattern can be important ways in which risk is reduced. This is dependent on the driver having insight about any impairment and being aware that they are becoming impaired. They need to act, either by avoiding driving when impaired or adapting their pattern of driving to ensure that it is within their capabilities.

Vehicle type

There are significant differences in the consequences of a dangerous incident for different types of vehicle (Table 2.3).

- *Large goods vehicles* have different performance profiles from cars in terms of braking, acceleration and steering, especially on wet roads. Their greater mass means that they have a greater potential than cars for damage to other road users. They may also carry dangerous loads.
- *Vans* are intermediate in performance profile between cars and large goods vehicles.

- *Buses and coaches*, because of their mass and performance, can also cause more consequential damage than cars. They can injure fare-paying passengers, who may have higher expectations of safety than a car passenger. In urban areas buses also will regularly be pointing at groups of passengers waiting to board at bus stops; loss of control in this situation has led to multiple fatalities. However, the passenger risks from bus and coach travel are far lower than those for car journeys.
- *Minibuses* fall between cars and larger vehicles in terms of performance, passenger risk and accident consequences. They are often driven by volunteers.
- *Taxis*, while no larger than cars, have to meet passenger expectations for driver fitness and for safety, both in terms of the vehicle and the driver's credentials.
- *Emergency vehicles* need to be able to travel at high speeds under difficult circumstances and so pose a high risk of accidents, which are partially mitigated by a high standard of driver training.
- The pattern of accident risk and consequential damage from *workplace vehicles* is very variable. Some, like forklift trucks, may be used in congested and peopled areas and have special issues of visibility when carrying loads. Others may

Table 2.3
Injury risks for different types of vehicle. Fatal and serious casualty rates per 100 million vehicle kilometres in Great Britain, 2004.[17]

	Drivers/riders	All casualties*
Cycles	60	62
Two-wheeled motor vehicles	121	138
Cars	2.6	7
Buses/coaches	0.9	26
Light goods vehicle	0.8	4
Heavy goods vehicle (>7.5 tonnes)	1.2	8

*These include all casualties from accidents (drivers, passengers, other road users, bystanders). There is some double counting where accidents involve more than one type of vehicle.

work on unstable ground in construction sites, while massive items of plant have the scope for causing large-scale damage from their mass.

- *Motorcycle* users are at very high personal risk and may injure others.
- Users of *bicycles, horses and power-assisted chairs and buggies*, none of which are regulated in terms of their capabilities, are all at risk from other road users while being relatively minor causes of risk to others.

Given these variables there is a wide range of training and competency requirements for drivers. Commonly there is also a more stringent medical assessment process, with higher standards for drivers of large vehicles and for those carrying fare-paying passengers. Responsibility for worksite and emergency vehicles and the fitness criteria to be met usually lies with the employer or the site operator.

Road and vehicle safety measures

There are differential risks for different classes of road, with motorways being the safest per mile travelled, and urban A and rural non-A roads being the most dangerous (Table 2.4).

Safety-related road improvements can benefit all users, but aspects such as better lighting and clearer signing will, in particular, help the older driver and others with visual problems. Many of the measures taken to segregate cyclists and pedestrians will also reduce the consequences of any incident associated with loss of control from driver impairment.

Table 2.4
Killed or seriously injured casualty rates: by road type per 100 million vehicle kilometres in Great Britain, 2004.[18]

Urban A road	8.68
Urban other	7.86
Rural A road	4.82
Rural other	8.43
Motorway	1.08

The mechanical reliability, warning systems and crashworthiness of vehicles have improved greatly in recent years. Risks to pedestrians from vehicle impact have been reduced by design and by prohibiting dangerous accessories like bull/roo bars. The profiles of some vehicles are inherently more dangerous than others.[19] In particular, the front profile of most cars is such that on impact a pedestrian will be lifted over the bonnet, while the higher profile of sports utility and other vehicles with high ground clearance is such that the pedestrian is likely to go under the vehicle and sustain more severe injuries.

Restraint of occupants by seat belts and airbags has also reduced the damage on impact. It is important that they are correctly fitted and worn.[20] Some drivers, eg those with stomas or painful lesions on their chest or abdomen, may find belts painful, and there are arrangements for medical practitioners to grant exemption by issuing a form that the driver must carry.[21] (Blank medical exemption certificates [called 'Certificates of Exemption from Compulsory Seat Belt Wearing'] are available to doctors only from the NHS distribution system, tel: 0870 155 5455.) However, it is preferable to modify the seat belt wherever possible, and details of suppliers of modifications are available via the Department for Transport's Mobility Advice and Information Service[22] or from other mobility centres (see p. 47).

For riders, protective clothing, such as a helmet and abrasion-resistant garments, play a part in risk reduction in the absence of the external barrier to impact provided by a vehicle body.

International comparisons

Road conditions vary widely worldwide, but even in the European Union there are major differences in injury frequency, with Scandinavia, the Netherlands and the UK among the countries with the lowest rates of fatal road crashes (Figure 2.3).[23]

The frequency of road crashes is almost always higher in the developing world than in more

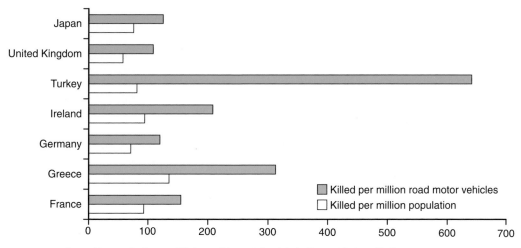

Source: European Conference of Ministers of Transport: Trends in the Transport Sector p.44–45

Figure 2.3
Selected international fatality rates.[23]

affluent countries, and road casualties are an even more major call on limited health and social care budget. For the traveller to the developing world an injury from a road crash is almost always the most common form of serious harm that can arise.

Consequences of crash-related injuries

There are continuing political tensions about the restrictions placed on drivers in the interests of road safety. This is because of an inherent difference of views between those who wish to drive as they choose and those who have suffered injury or bereavement or who are responsible for the care of casualties. In the case of health-related impairment and the risk of crashes this is further complicated by the sometimes conflicting roles of clinicians. They may wish to prevent casualties on the roads but may also need to act as advocates for their patients who wish to continue driving. They may be promoters of healthier lifestyles less dependent on vehicle use, but will often be regular drivers themselves! Neither these

conflicts nor the harm from injury is the focus of this book but the following points are worth noting.

- Injuries and death from road crashes are a major cause of disability in the young.
- Child pedestrians are vulnerable on urban roads. The UK rates for child pedestrian accidents are disproportionately high when compared with other parts of north western Europe.
- Young cyclists are similarly at risk.
- Head injury, especially in cyclists and motorcyclists, is a major cause of severe long-term disability, partially prevented by helmets.
- More frequent but less serious road injuries lead to loss of time from work.
- Some consequences of crashes, such as 'whiplash' injury to the neck, may be the subject of litigation to seek compensation. The effects of the legal process and the need to show disability may stand in the way of early recovery.

Because of the young age distribution of fatal injuries from road crashes, these injuries make a disproportionate contribution to loss of years from life as compared to most forms of ill-health which predominate in later life. The current economic estimates used to evaluate the value of preventative measures are: fatal £1.4m, seriously injured £156k, slightly injured £12k.[24] These estimates include allowances for health costs, for loss of earnings and for costs of care for dependants.

Summary

- For most road crashes the major contributor is the driver; crashes caused by road conditions and vehicle defects are much less common.

- Several techniques can be used to assess the road safety risks from health-related impairment. All have limitations.

- Other causes of driver impairment can interact with medical conditions to cause accidents.

- The consequences of a crash differ with vehicle type and depend on the vulnerability of those injured.

- Injuries from road crashes are an important cause of morbidity and mortality.

- Road and vehicle design can reduce risk.

References

1. Taylor J, ed. *Medical Aspects of Fitness to Drive*. Medical Commission on Accident Prevention, 1995.

2. Sabey BE, Staughton GC. Interacting roles of road, environment, vehicle and road user accidents. Fifth International Conference of the International Association of Accident and Traffic Medicine, London, 1975.

3. Treat JR, *et al. Trilevel Study of Cause of Traffic Accidents*. Report No. DOT-034-3-5-35-77(TAC). Indiana University, 1988.

4. Mosedale J, Purdy A, Clarkson E. *Contributory Factors to Road Accidents. Transport Statistics: Road Safety*. London: HMSO, 2004. www.dft.gov.uk/stellent/groups/ dft_rdsafety/documents/divisionhomepage/030263.hcsp

5. Grattan E, Jeffcoate GO. Medical factors and road accidents. *BMJ* 1968; **1**: 75.

6. Vernon DD, Diller EM, Cook LJ, *et al*. Evaluating the crash and citation rates of Utah drivers licensed with medical conditions, 1992–1996. *Accid Anal Prev* 2002; **34**: 237–246.

7. *Road Casualties Great Britain – 2004 Annual Report*. London: Department for Transport, 2004: 60. www.dft.gov.uk/stellent/groups/dft_control/documents/ contentservertemplate/dft_index.hcst?n=14456&l=5

8. Charlton J, *et al. Influence of Chronic Illness on Crash Involvement of Motor Vehicle Drivers*. Report No. 213. Accident Research Centre, Monash University, 2004. www.monash.edu.au/muarc/reports/muarc213.pdf

9. Dobbs BM. *Medical Conditions and Driving: A Review of the Literature 1960–2000*. DOT HS 809 690. Washington DC: National Highway Transportation Safety Administration, 2005. www.nhtsa.dot.gov/people/injury/research/ MedicalConditions_Driving.pdf

10. *Safe Mobility for Older Drivers: Notebook*. DOT HS 808 853. Washington DC: National Highway Transportation Safety Administration, 1999. www.nhtsa.dot.gov/people/injury/ olddrive/safe/index.htm

11. *Road Casualties Great Britain 2004*. London: Department for Transport, 2004: 27. www.dft.gov.uk/stellent/groups/dft_transstats/ documents/page/dft_transstats_041285.pdf

12. Evans L. *Traffic Safety and the Driver*. New York: Van Nostrand Reinhold, 1991: 162–191.

13. Horne J, Reyner L. *Driver sleepiness*. Road Safety Research Report 21. London: Department for Transport, 2001. www.dft.gov.uk/stellent/groups/dft_rdsafety/documents/ page/dft_rdsafety_504598.hcsp

14. Evans L. *Traffic Safety and the Driver*. New York: Van Nostrand Reinhold, 1991: 133–161.

15. Zuckerman M. *Behavioural Expressions and Biosocial Bases of Sensation Seeking*. Cambridge: Cambridge University Press, 1994.

16. *Road Casualties in Great Britain 2004*. London: Department for Transport, 2005: 60–61

17. *Road Casualties in Great Britain: 2004 Annual Report*. London: Department for Transport, 2004: 60–61 (with additional data from Department for Transport Statistics – Road Safety). www.dft.gov.uk/stellent/groups/dft_transstats/ documents/page/dft_transstats_041290.pdf

18. Unpublished data from Statistics Branch, Department for Transport, tabulated on request.

19. Simms C, O'Neill D. Sports utility vehicles and older pedestrians. *BMJ* 2005; **331**: 787–788.

20. Department for Transport. *Seat Belts and Child Restraints*. (T/INF/251) London: Department for Transport, 2005. www.thinkroadsafety.gov.uk/advice/seatbelts.htm

21. *Medical Exemption form Compulsory Seat Belt Wearing: Guidance for Medical Practitioners*. London: Department for Environment, Transport and the Regions, 1999. (Available from Department for Transport)

22. www.dft.gov.uk/stellent/groups/dft_mobility/ documents/page/dft_mobility_503255.hcsp

23. European Conference of Ministers of Transport. *Trends in*

the Transport Sector: 44–45.
www.cemt.org/events/JustPub/justTrends.htm

24. Department for Transport. Highways Economic Note 1:
2004. www.dft.gov.uk/stellent/groups/dft_rdsafety/
documents/page/dft_rdsafety_610642.hcsp

3. Who does what?

The regulatory framework, the driver and the DVLA
Other groups with responsibilities

The wide range of health-related impairments influencing fitness to drive mean that there is a very wide range of responsibilities for action. This chapter identifies what these are and how they interact with each other. The responsibilities described relate to road safety law in Great Britain, where the Driver and Vehicle Licensing Agency (DVLA) is the licensing authority. Arrangements in Northern Ireland are almost identical. Some comparisons with other countries are also noted.

The regulatory framework, the driver and the DVLA

The law and regulations

As driving on public roads requires a licence, the actions of all those involved are set by the arrangements for licensing and the obligations that these place on each party. The applicant for a licence, usually at first a provisional one when learning to drive is started, accepts a set of conditions and obligations, such as the need to pass the driving test and to drive in a safe and courteous manner, as described in the *Highway Code*.[1] Applicants also have obligations related to their health:

- They must not drive while impaired by alcohol or drugs, the latter including prescription and over-the-counter medications.

- In some circumstances they need to notify the DVLA of medical conditions. The DVLA acts as the licensing authority on behalf of the Secretary of State for Transport, who is responsible in legislation. These medical conditions are prescribed by law.

— On application for a licence or when renewing a licence (DVLA application forms: D1 – ordinary licence, D2 – large goods vehicle/passenger carrying vehicle; renewals: D46, D47) the applicant completes a declaration stating whether they are suffering or have suffered from any of a series of listed impairing medical conditions (see p. 23). Relevant disabilities include some that are prescribed (Road Traffic Act Section 92 [1]). They also include any other disability likely to cause the driving of a vehicle to be a source of danger to the public. A prospective disability is one that is not relevant at the time of licence issue or notification but that may become relevant later because it is intermittent or progressive.

— The licence holder must notify the DVLA if they become aware that they are suffering from a relevant or prospective disability, either a new one or an old one that has become more acute. An exception is made if the disability is new and they have reasonable grounds for believing that its duration will not exceed three months (Road Traffic Act Section 94 [1]).

- In addition, the presence of a medical condition that interferes with driving is not necessarily a defence if charged with careless or dangerous driving, or with failing to be in a position to exercise proper control over a vehicle.

Licences are granted for a range of types of vehicle and there are, for example, different tests for car driving, motorcycling and driving large vehicles. In terms of health-related criteria there are two main licence categories; these are common throughout the European Union:

Group 1: cars, vans, etc less than 3.5 tonnes in weight or with up to eight passenger seats, for new licence holders, but less than 7.5 tonnes or up to 16 passenger seats for those issued with a licence before 1 January 1997. The same medical standards and responsibilities apply to motor bicycle and tricycle drivers. The category C1 applies to vehicles such as large vans and camper vans and medium-sized trucks of between 3.5 and 7.5 tonnes, while D1 is the category for minibuses with between 9 and 16 passenger seats.[2]

- In the UK the licensing of a car driver is entirely dependent on the driver's self-declaration of disability, with the exception of a simple vision test and any observations of a driving examiner at the time of test for new drivers.

- Medical information is only obtained where there is an indication to do so, normally after a declaration by the driver or because of a notification to the DVLA from someone else such as a relative, neighbour, health professional or the police.

Group 2: trucks and buses more than 3.5 tonnes in weight or with more than eight passenger seats for holders of new licences including those re-issued for medical reasons, but more than 7.5 tonnes or more than 16 passenger seats for those issued with a licence before 1 January 1997. There are requirements in addition to self-declaration which apply to holders of Group 2 licences.

- The medical criteria for granting a licence are more stringent because of the longer period normally spent driving and because of the more severe consequences of a large vehicle crash.

- Issue of the licence requires the applicant to submit a standardized report of a medical assessment (Form D4). The assessment can be done by any doctor but is normally done by the individual's general practitioner, who will have access to their medical records. The driver or their employer is responsible for the cost of

providing this report. At present (under discussion in the European Union) this medical report must be submitted by the driver when first licensed, not normally before 21 years of age, every five years from 45 to 65 years, and thereafter annually.

- A Group 2 driver will also hold a Group 1 licence and hence they have an obligation to declare any new disability, but this will be assessed by the DVLA in relation to the Group 2 standards as well as those for Group 1.

These legal requirements form the basis for the more detailed criteria used by the DVLA when making decisions on medical aspects of licensing. The requirements are summarized as a reminder to drivers when they apply or re-apply for a licence. In turn they determine what advice from health professionals is needed, at least for the longer term and for more seriously impairing conditions that enter the licensing framework.

The following offences under the Road Traffic Act 1988 can be applied to individuals who drive while unfit:

- driving after making a false declaration as to physical fitness: S 92 (10)

- failing to notify the Secretary of State of onset or deterioration of disability: S 94 (3)

- driving after such a failure

- driving with uncorrected defective eyesight or refusing to submit to a test of eyesight: S 96

- making a false statement to obtain a driving licence or certificate of insurance: S 174.

Failure to inform the DVLA of a notifiable medical condition is punishable by a licence endorsement and could result in disqualification. A fine of up to £1000 can also be imposed. Knowingly making a false statement for the purpose of obtaining a licence may result in up to two years' imprisonment.

Prescribed disabilities

Disabilities that are prescribed by regulations (Motor Vehicles [Driving Licence] Regulations 1999 Part 4, paras 70–72) made under the Road Traffic Act (Section 92) (paraphrased) are as follows.

For a person who holds a Group 1 or Group 2 licence:

a) *epilepsy* (defined for Group 1 as free of an attack for one year or attacks only while asleep for more than three years. For Group 2 as 10 years free of attacks without requiring any medication to treat epilepsy)

b) *severe mental disorder* (includes mental illness, arrested or incomplete development of the mind, psychopathic disorder and severe impairment of intelligence or social functioning)

c) liability to *sudden attacks of disabling giddiness or fainting* which are caused by any disorder or defect of the heart as a result of which the applicant for the licence or, as the case may be, the holder of the licence has a device implanted in their body, being a device which, by operating on the heart so as to regulate its action, is designed to correct the disorder or defect. (Driving may be allowed if the person is unlikely to be a source of danger to the public and if they are receiving regular medical supervision from a cardiologist.)

d) liability to *sudden attacks of disabling giddiness or fainting*, other than attacks falling within paragraph 1 (c)

e) absence, deformity or non-progressive *loss of the use of one or more limbs or parts of limbs*.

For a person who holds a Group 1 licence:

f) *inability to read in good daylight* (with the aid of corrective lenses if necessary) a registration plate fixed to a motor vehicle and containing letters and figures 79.4 mm high at a distance of 20.5 m (12.3 m in the case of an applicant for a licence for a pedestrian-guided vehicle such as a motor mower).

Additionally for a Group 2 licence:

g) *visual acuity*: less than 6/9 in the better eye, 6/12 in the worse eye – corrected. Uncorrected less than 3/60 in both eyes. There are some concessions for those who gained a Group 2 licence when the standards were different.

h) *diabetes requiring insulin treatment*. (There are some concessions, including drivers who were licensed while on insulin some while ago, or who drive goods vehicles between 3.5 and 7.5 tonnes, who are under regular surveillance by a diabetologist and who demonstrate good control, free from hypoglycaemic episodes.)

The driver

The driver, as a condition of their licence, is personally responsible for ensuring that they are fit to drive, refraining from driving if they are not and in some circumstances informing the DVLA as the licensing authority. In addition they must not be impaired to drive by alcohol or drugs. This includes prescribed or over the counter medication. Their condition must not prevent control of the vehicle or lead to careless or dangerous driving.

Any driver will face conflicting pressures between the need for mobility and their perception of their present state of capability. This perception will be based on:

- subjective feelings, eg of tiredness or of debility from, say, a viral infection
- response to indicators of impairment, eg inebriation from alcohol use or tiredness from lack of sleep
- noting if they are unusually clumsy or error prone
- advice given by health professionals or by warning labels on medication
- their knowledge and understanding of any risks of sudden incapacity associated with their current state of health.

There are also obligations on all drivers that form part of the licence conditions – see above.

The DVLA advises drivers that: 'You *must* tell the DVLA if you have ever had or currently suffer from any of these conditions:[3]

- epilepsy
- fit(s) or blackouts
- repeated attacks of sudden disabling giddiness
- diabetes controlled by insulin
- diabetes controlled by tablets
- an implanted cardiac pacemaker
- an implanted cardiac defibrillator (ICD)
- angina (heart pain) which is easily brought on by driving
- persistent alcohol misuse or dependency
- persistent drug use or dependency
- Parkinson's disease
- narcolepsy or sleep apnoea syndrome
- stroke, with any symptoms lasting longer than one month, recurrent 'mini-strokes' or transient ischaemic attacks (TIAs)
- any type of brain surgery, severe head injury involving in-patient treatment, or brain tumour
- any other chronic neurological condition
- a serious problem with memory or episodes of confusion
- severe learning disability

- serious psychiatric illness or mental ill-health
- total loss of sight in one eye
- any condition affecting both eyes, or the remaining eye if one eye only (excluding short/long sight or colour blindness)
- any condition affecting your visual field
- any persistent limb problem which requires your driving to be restricted to certain types of vehicles or those with adapted controls.

There are extra rules for larger vehicles: 'As well as those medical conditions already stated, you also need to notify the DVLA about:

- visual problems affecting either eye
- angina or other heart condition, or heart operation
- any form of stroke, including TIA.

If you want to drive lorries or buses you must not have a liability to epileptic seizures.

Insulin-treated diabetics may not drive large vehicles unless:

- they held a licence to drive lorries or buses on 1 April 1991, and
- the Traffic Commissioner who issued the licence or in whose area they lived, was aware of the insulin treatment before January 1991.'

Whenever a licence holder becomes aware that they are suffering from a notifiable disability they must notify the DVLA, which has powers to require an individual:

- to give consent for their doctors and specialists to provide medical reports
- to attend a doctor or other assessor, such as an optometrist, to determine if they are fit to drive.

Refusal to do so can be sufficient grounds to turn down an application or revoke a licence. The driver has the option of voluntarily surrendering their licence, in which case further medical enquiries will not be made until such time as they request that it is re-instituted.

This is rather different from the normal approach to medical consent, because failure to give it has inevitable consequences. This is

because noncompliance is treated in the same way as having a disability that bars an individual from driving.

In terms of the Human Rights Act 1998, holding a driving licence is neither an absolute right, nor is it a privilege that can be taken away without reason. It is what is termed a qualified right (Article 8: private life. Protocol 1, Article 1: enjoyment of property). Interference with qualified rights is permissible only if what is done meets certain conditions:

- it has its basis in law
- it is necessary in a democratic society, ie:
  —fulfils a pressing social need
  —pursues a legitimate aim
  —is proportionate to the aims being pursued, eg the protection of public health or order.

Thus the fair application of statutory standards to prevent death and injury on the roads meets the required criteria.

Any system that relies on self-declaration is likely to suffer from a degree of under-reporting, particularly when declaration can result in loss of a driving licence. There have not been any recent studies on the proportion of cases of conditions that require notification which have been declared to the DVLA. However, unpublished results comparing population incidence rates of conditions listed as requiring declaration with the number of cases notified to the DVLA suggest that failure to declare is not uncommon.

The DVLA

The Driver and Vehicle Licensing Agency in Swansea is an agency of the Department for Transport. The agency issues all driving licences for Great Britain on behalf of the Secretary of State. Northern Ireland has a separate licensing authority which has very similar duties and standards. The Medical Group at DVLA assesses medical aspects of fitness.[4] The provisions of the Road Traffic Act 1988 and associated regulations form the basis for decision-taking and these are supplemented by Medical Standards of Fitness to Drive. These standards are published in the *At A Glance Guide*.[5] These standards are used by the agency for taking decisions. Standards for common medical conditions, as they apply to Group 1 and Group 2 drivers, are listed and there is additional background information on some of the more

complex ones. The standards are updated regularly based on advice from the Secretary of State's Honorary Medical Panels on Fitness to Drive and from other sources of expertise. These panels cover: heart disease, neurology, diabetes, vision, mental health, and drug and alcohol problems. Details of membership, annual reports of the panels and recent minutes are available.[6,7] Patients may sometimes be aware of the discussions about standards which are in progress from these sources.

The medical group at the DVLA handled about 400 000 Group 1 cases and 67 000 Group 2 cases in 2004. Of these 86% were granted, or continued to hold, a licence. Two hundred administrative and 17 medical staff are members of the Medical Group. The most common groups of conditions dealt with are: diabetes, where many licences are of limited duration; neurological, including epilepsy; cardiovascular problems, particularly in Group 2 drivers; vision; and alcohol and drug misuse.

The DVLA receives notifications concerning fitness to drive from a range of sources (Table 3.1). The majority come from drivers themselves but family members, neighbours, the police and health professionals may also provide information.

Notifications to the DVLA of a possible disabling condition, as well as the periodic medical examination reports on Group 2 drivers, are assessed using a staged process:

1. The information provided by the notifier is evaluated.

Table 3.1
Health-related notifications to the DVLA, 2004. Reproduced with permission.

Total	120 782 (most from drivers themselves)
Police	3 512 (usually following an accident or incident)
Driving Standards Agency	1 062 (from driving test centres)
Courts	45 (excluding high-risk offenders scheme)
Anonymous	18
Doctors	2 218
Others	11 998 (often colleagues or family members)

2. Many reported conditions are reviewed according to standing instructions and a licence issued or revoked on this basis.

3. More detailed information may be sought from the driver or their medical advisers. In the first instance this is usually done using standard questionnaires which seek information rather than opinion.

4. Sometimes additional investigations or consultations are required, especially for Group 2 drivers. In most cases the DVLA pays a fee for any additional information or investigation it requests and this is an overhead covered by the standard licence fee paid by all drivers.

5. Cases where there is uncertainty or where multiple conditions are present are referred to a DVLA medical adviser for assessment based on the reports provided or on additional information the adviser obtains from clinicians. Advisers work to the DVLA standards but are able to take a better informed view in complex cases, in particular by considering, if more than one medical condition is notified, which are the critical ones, and whether any interactions can be expected between them which could affect risk. This aspect of the work is increasing in volume as the number of older drivers with complex patterns of pathology increases.

6. Some forms of stable impairment require individual assessment and at times advice on driving or re-training to manage a new disability or modification to a vehicle. The DVLA can refer such cases to a mobility centre for an assessment (see p. 47).

7. A very small proportion of cases are reviewed by the relevant medical panel, either because of their difficulty or because they relate to a topic where it is considered that the standards may need to be revised. The latter often result from developments in diagnostic methods or treatment not previously encountered by the DVLA.

When there is sufficient information, the licence will be issued, possibly with a restricted duration or limited to a specially modified vehicle. However, in a small proportion of cases it is refused or revoked. The vast majority of notifications to the DVLA do not result in loss of licence, and health professionals should bring this to the attention of anyone they advise to notify.

If a licence is refused or revoked, the applicant has a right of appeal to a magistrate's court in England and Wales or to a sheriff's court in Scotland (Table 3.2).

There will a period between notification to the DVLA and a decision on the continuation or revocation of an existing licence. During this period the driver remains formally entitled to drive and it is their decision, based on medical advice, as to whether or not they are fit to do so. Hence the clinician has a key role in giving the driver clear and valid advice on whether or not they should drive prior to the DVLA's decision.

The DVLA is able to advise both drivers and clinicians on fitness to drive. Drivers should contact the DVLA helpline (tel: 0870 600 0301; email eftd@dvla.gsi.gov.uk). One of the medical advisers will be available to answer questions from clinicians during working hours. There is also an email enquiry service for clinicians linked to the *At A Glance* website. (Medical professionals only may contact DVLA medical staff on 01792 761119 [Northern Ireland: 028 703 41369] or medadviser.dvla@gtnet.gov.uk.)

Table 3.2

Appeals on DVLA medical licensing decisions over four years between 2000 and 2004.* Reproduced with permission.

Summons	801
Withdrawn before hearing	693
Full hearing	108
Dismissed	100
Upheld	8

*Many of the appeals were concerned with licensing decisions about alcohol misuse or dependency.

Other groups with responsibilities

Suppliers of impairing products

The two most common categories of impairing product are alcohol and medications. Few alcoholic products bear direct warnings, although most now carry either information on the strength of the beverage or on how much represents a unit of consumption. The latter can, as with unmeasured home-poured alcoholic drinks, be confusing if the size of a measure is not standard or if, as with premium lagers and strong ciders, the strength differs from the norm for that type of beverage. General information on drink and driving comes through a variety of channels. The driver's behaviour is influenced both by social norms about drinking and driving and the risk of loss of licence if they are tested (see Chapter 14).

Medications carry warnings on driving where relevant. These may be on the pharmacist's label, on the packet or in the patient information leaflet. Labelling may need to be supplemented by personal advice from the pharmacist or other supplier on the medication's effects on driving and other safety-critical tasks (see Chapter 13).

The health professional

Any clinician has a duty to advise their patient of likely impairments to driving.[8] The nature of this will depend on their practice and the legal framework in the country in which they are practising.

- *Medical practitioners* will encounter a wide range of impairments determined by the practitioner's speciality and the age group of patients seen.[9]
- The *pharmacist* in their prescribing role will be largely concerned with medications but may also be called on to advise more widely.
- The *optometrist* will focus on visual limitations, including the inherent ones of the patient's eyes, the need to take care when adapting to new lenses or types of correction, and the short-term limitations following the use of ocular medications.
- *Physiotherapists and practitioners using manipulation* are likely to need to advise on pain or strength-related musculoskeletal limitations.
- *Complementary and alternative therapists* may induce deep relaxation which can impair driving performance for brief periods afterwards.
- The use of *sedatives, local or general anaesthetics* as adjuncts to medical or dental treatment will also call for specific advice. This needs to be given before the patient attends for a planned procedure so that they do not drive to the appointment and thus have to drive home afterwards.

Specific aspects of the clinical consultation are covered in Chapter 5. All groups of health professionals are accountable to their professional bodies for the conduct of their practice. Advice on fitness to drive forms a part of this practice and can lead to conflict between patient advocacy and public safety.

The driver agrees to a set of conditions, including notification of impairing illness, when the licence is issued. There is scope for a driver to be unaware of or to ignore illness and associated impairment. It is good practice for any health professional to give a driver definite instructions about any likely risk of impairment, especially when pressure to keep the patient driving, even if they are impaired, can be anticipated.

Group 2 drivers will request medical assessments and completion of DVLA form D4 on application for and renewal of the licence.

The DVLA may request information when a licence is issued or at other times to assist its investigations on fitness to hold a licence. The driver making the request can be charged a fee. The DVLA has specified fees for any requests it makes. Employers, insurers and others may request medical reports in relation to fitness to drive.

The Department for Transport

The DVLA is responsible for licensing, while its parent department, working with other bodies such as the police and highway authorities, is responsible for wider aspects of driver performance and road safety. In particular, the Department for Transport is responsible for:

- the measures taken to reduce the risks from non-health-related driver impairment, eg as a consequence of alcohol or drug use and abuse
- liaison with medicines regulatory bodies about testing and labelling in relation to driving performance
- behavioural and cognitive aspects of driving safety, especially as they relate to different groups of drivers, such as the young and the old
- the performance, risks and safety of other road users, such as child and adult pedestrians, cyclists, horse riders and powered wheelchair and buggy drivers
- the safety and human factor aspects of the design and operational standards for vehicles and roads
- maintaining mobility by meeting the special needs of disabled drivers, other road users and pedestrians, by improving access to all forms of transport and by assessment of individuals to ensure that the effects of any disability on outdoor mobility are minimized
- managing research programmes supporting these topics and the medical standards for driving.[10–12]

The police

Traffic safety and the detection of motoring offences form a large part of the duties of police forces. It is frequently the judgement of a police officer, either when observing poor driving performance or after an accident, which leads to an investigation of driving impairment. Their most direct concerns are in connection with road traffic offences associated with driver behaviour and the impairing effects of alcohol, drug misuse and fatigue. Where they suspect

alcohol-related impairment they use roadside tests for breath alcohol (see Chapter 14). For suspected impairment from drugs they may require a 'field impairment test' which assesses performance capabilities that are likely to identify drug-related impairment. Soon these could be supplemented by roadside drug screening devices. Officers may sometimes check a driver's vision using the number plate test (p. 23, box).

In cases where impairment needs to be assessed, forensic medical examiners assist the police by taking blood samples when they consider, after a clinical examination, that a condition due to alcohol or drugs is present. Should police investigation of poor driving performance or an accident indicate that there may be health-related impairment, this may lead to a caution where the driver is recommended to seek advice on their fitness to drive, to referral to the DVLA – especially where there is a pre-existing medical condition that may have contributed to an incident – or more rarely to a prosecution for driving while unfit to do so.

The European Union

The UK driving licence is valid across the European Union (EU), while licences issued in other member states are valid in the UK. The EC Driving Licence Directive[13] includes procedures for granting licences, a common classification of vehicles for licensing, the format of the licence and an annex listing medical standards. All of these are used as the basis for British and other national standards. The medical standards represent minimum requirements and are not as specific as those in most member states. Member states are accountable to the EU for the ways in which they implement directives, but the means by which compliance with medical standards is assessed is a matter for each member. There are considerable differences in approach.

- Licensing may be local, at municipal or county level or, as in Great Britain, a national responsibility.
- For Group 1 drivers, self-declaration or

regular medical surveillance, with or without self-declaration, may form the basis for decisions.

- Licences may be renewed at different intervals and there are also variations in whether the decision on health-related impairment at re-licensing depends on self-declaration or some form of health check.
- The licensing authority may have its own medical advisers to take decisions or it may use the patient's clinician, a network of approved doctors or a driving fitness assessment centre.
- The detail of tests used may differ; thus, Britain is unusual in using its large typeface number plates rather than the standard optometrist's acuity measures for vision assessment.
- There may be variations in the way in which discretion is exercised. For example, some of the standards allow for 'exceptional cases', the meaning of which, eg in relation to Group 2 drivers on insulin, can be interpreted in a variety of ways. Discretion may also be implicit rather than stated. For example, a system such as Britain's, which relies on review of submitted reports, may pay less attention to an intuitive view of a driver's attitude to risk than one involving clinical examination. While a doctor who is also the driver's clinician may to an extent act as a patient's advocate rather than as a medical examiner, they will, unlike a doctor approved to do driver medicals, have full access to medical records. This should avoid non-disclosure of past ill-health.
- Some states place a duty on all doctors to inform the licensing authority in the event of certain diagnoses, such as epilepsy, or any condition likely to impair driving. This clarifies the doctor's position but possibly at the expense of the clinical relationship, and hence it may inhibit diagnosis and management of ill-health.
- The EU has a research programme on road safety which includes projects assessing fitness to drive.[14]

There is very little evaluation of the consequences of these differences among EU member states, either in terms of maintaining a driver's mobility or in relation to driving performance and accidents.

Beyond the EU the driving standards for a number of countries are accessible on the internet.[15,16] Many similarities are apparent, but the boundaries vary between what levels of impairment are and are not acceptable, often between state/provincial jurisdictions in the same federal country.

Some countries, such as the USA, Canada and Australia, have very well developed programmes for topics such as the assessment of the older driver. These include high-quality information resources that are directed at health professionals (see Appendix 1).

Driver assessment centres

A national network of mobility assessment centres working to broadly similar standards is available to evaluate the performance of drivers with stable impairments and to advise the driver, clinicians or the licensing authority on whether they can drive safely and on whether any re-training, vehicle modifications or limits to driving are recommended (see p. 47). Some local and county road safety units provide rather simpler assessments which are usually geared to helping drivers, mainly elderly ones, to make sound decisions about whether they should continue to drive.

The assessment centres work closely with the suppliers and modifiers of vehicles for those with special needs. The 'Motability' scheme provides leasing and other financial arrangements for those drivers who qualify for assistance with the purchase of vehicles because of their disabilities (see p. 49).

Insurers

Insurers now accept that if an individual is fit to hold a licence in the eyes of the DVLA then they are eligible for motor insurance. Thus they do not make any separate assessment of fitness but will, if notified of an illness, usually advise the driver to inform the DVLA of the date of diagnosis, treatment and stability of the condition.

If a driver has not declared a notifiable condition to the DVLA of which they are aware, then their insurance cover may be formally invalid. Health professionals, when advising drivers to declare a disability to the DVLA, should make them aware that if they fail to do so then their motor insurance could be invalid. Even those who do not personally hold insurance for a car should be advised about this risk if they have a condition where declaration to the DVLA is indicated, as any policy under which they are driving will also be invalid if they are the driver at the time of an accident. In the event of an accident, the driver can be held personally liable for the costs of any damage done, although if they do not have sufficient assets to pay third-party costs (claims for injury or loss of earnings in others, for damage to other cars or to property) these may be met under the arrangements for accidents by uninsured drivers. Failure to have third-party insurance when driving, like driving while unlicensed, is a criminal offence.

Insurers load premiums for those with poor accident records, for high-risk groups such as the young driver, and for those with a record of alcohol-related or other driving offences. They used to charge higher premiums for some forms of disability and chronic illness but no longer do so, both because of their own claims experience, which indicates no excess accident risk, and also to be in accord with disability discrimination legislation.

Employers and organizations using volunteer drivers

Employers and those using volunteer drivers may need to consider fitness to drive as part of the risk assessment required under health and safety law or because of concerns about public liability. Their assessment may indicate that fitness standards over and above those of the Road Traffic Act 1988, and as a consequence

those applied by the DVLA, are appropriate for driving on public roads. Examples include emergency service drivers in the police, fire, ambulance and coastguard services (see Chapter 7).

Worksites which are not public highways have special risks even for normal road vehicles, eg airside driving at airports. Many specialized vehicles such as forklift trucks, tractors and cranes are used in workplaces. The vehicle and the working environment in which it is used (eg a farm, construction site or cold store) may create novel patterns of risk and thus require an assessment of fitness to drive which is based on the risks and job requirements identified in the employer's health and safety risk assessment (see p. 64).

Local authorities

In addition to their role as employers, local authorities are responsible for licensing taxi drivers. These licences are issued locally, as decisions on the number of licences, the conduct of each individual applying and their continuing suitability to hold a licence all form part of the process. As the DVLA issues licences in terms of vehicle size and not use, Group 1 standards are the legal minimum for taxi driving. The majority of taxi licensing authorities use the Group 2 standards as the basis for acceptance because of the public safety implications of health-related impairment in a driver who carries passengers for financial reward (see p. 64).

County authorities are responsible for local roads and road safety. Some run programmes and campaigns concerned with fitness to drive, providing drivers, particularly older ones, with advice and opportunities for assessment.

Medical charities

A number of the larger associations concerned with campaigning and research into particular diseases, eg The British Heart Foundation, Diabetes UK and the epilepsy associations, produce excellent guidance on driving for their members and for other sufferers as well as for health professionals (see Chapters 10–21). They also campaign and undertake case work to ensure that their members are fairly handled in terms of the assessment of fitness to drive, and to try and secure changes to the criteria used.

The international scientific community

While the fitness criteria used by different national regulators may differ in detail, the evidence on which they should be based is in large measure international. At regional level, eg in the EU, there are co-ordinated research programmes and scientific working groups. Internationally the OECD and the WHO have taken initiatives on fitness to drive. A number of scientific and professional associations have sections concerned with fitness to drive. There are also conferences and symposia, most notably the International Association of Traffic Medicine (www.trafficmedicine.org), the International Council on Alcohol, Drugs and Traffic Safety (www.icadts.org), and Vision in Vehicles. The latter combines many disciplines concerned with ergonomics, road and vehicle design and driver behaviour, as well as with medical aspects of vision.[17]

References

1. Driving Standards Agency. *Highway Code*. London: The Stationery Office.

2. *Driving Licence Information*. DVLA leaflet INS57P. Swansea: DVLA. www.direct.gov.uk/motoring

3. *What You Need to Know about Driving Licences*, DVLA leaflet D100, p 29. (12/05). Swansea: DVLA. www.dvla.gov.uk/forms/pdf/D100.pdf

4. *Customer Service Guide for Drivers with Medical Conditions*. Inf. 94. Swansea: DVLA, 2003.

5. Drivers Medical Group. *At a Glance Guide to Medical Standards of Fitness to Drive*. Swansea: DVLA. (Updated six-monthly.) www.dvla.gov.uk/at_a_glance/content.htm

6. Medical Panel members: www.dvla.gov.uk/drivers/medical/panel_members.htm

7. Medical panel meetings, minutes and reports: www.dvla.gov.uk/drivers/medical/agenda_main.htm

8. Nunez VA, Giddins GEB. 'Doctor, when can I drive?': an update on the medico-legal aspects of driving following an injury or operation. *Injury* 2004; **35**: 888–890.

9. Odell M. Assessing fitness to drive. *Aust Fam Phys* 2005; **34**: 359–362, 475–477.

10. Department for Transport Road Safety Research Reports. www.dft.gov.uk/stellent/groups/dft_rdsafety/documents/divisionhomepage/032513.hcsp

11. Department for Transport Medical Aspects of Fitness to Drive Reports index. www.dft.gov.uk/stellent/groups/dft_rdsafety/documents/divisionhomepage/030264.hcsp

12. Department for Transport Compendium of Current Research. www.dft.gov.uk/stellent/groups/dft_rdsafety/documents/divisionhomepage/032511.hcsp

13. Second EC Driver Licensing Directive (Directive 91/439/EEC).

14. Alvarez JF, del Rio MC, Fierro I *et al*. *Medical condition and fitness to drive; prospective analysis of the medical-psychological assessment of fitness to drive and accident risk*. Spain: Mata Digital, 2004.

15. *Assessing Fitness to Drive for Commercial and Private Vehicle Drivers*. Australia: Austroads Inc, 2003. www.austroads.com.au/aftd/downloads/AFTD_2003_FA_WEBREV1.pdf

16. *Medical Aspects of Fitness to Drive: A Guide for Medical Practitioners*. New Zealand: Land Transport Safety Authority, 2002. www.landtransport.govt.nz/licensing/docs/ltsa-medical-aspects.pdf

17. www.lboro.ac.uk/research/esri/applied-vision/projects/visioninvehicles/prevconf.html

4. Driving and the clinical consultation

Advice to drivers
Medical examiner function

Advice to drivers

The vast majority of adults, and hence patients, will be drivers (Table 4.1), although older females are less likely to hold a licence, and a proportion of older people will have given up driving. Almost all children will also expect to become drivers. Most of a health professional's contacts will be concerned with ill-health and the remedies for it. Hence assessment of and advice about fitness to drive will need to form part of the consultation if a newly presented condition or a change to an existing illness/disability or its treatment, in particular with medication, is likely to impair driving either temporarily or in the longer term.

Deciding whether a driver needs advice about fitness to drive requires the health professional to understand the capability requirements for driving and the conditions and treatments that may impair it. As a health professional you need to be able to give driving advice or know how

to direct patients to a competent source of advice. At times you will need additional information based on investigation or specialist expertise in order to give valid advice. Where this is needed, eg in assessing and correcting a visual problem, a referral for advice or treatment forms part of good professional practice. You should avoid making limited, sketchy or insecure recommendations about fitness to drive, as these may either over-restrict the driver or be too lenient and lead to a crash where the health professional's advice may be cited when issues of liability for injury or damage arise.

When clinical care is undertaken by a team, eg prior to discharge from inpatient treatment, the team leader should ensure that the responsibility for advising on driving is clearly allocated and that those giving such advice are competent to do so, document the advice given and ensure that others, such as the general practitioner involved in follow-up, are informed of it. Where a limited range of conditions is treated, eg in a fracture or diabetes clinic, it is often best to use standardized written advice. This can be explained to the patient by a member of the team who has this task as one of their responsibilities.

Evidence – health professionals and advice on fitness to drive

● The health professions are highly influential sources of advice on driving behaviour. A recent study ranked sources of

Table 4.1
Driving licence holders in Great Britain, 2004 by age group.[1]

	All aged 17+	17–20	21–29	30–39	40–49	50–59	60–69	70–79	80 and over	Estimated number of licence holders (millions)
All adults (%)	70	28	68	82	84	79	73	53	30	32.3
Men (%)	81	31	74	88	91	90	87	75	52	17.9
Women (%)	61	24	62	77	78	69	59	33	17	14.4

advice in terms of percentage ratings for being highly influential: GP 94%, optician 91%, police and courts 72%, the DVLA 52%, family 48%.[2]

- There is evidence that some groups of health professional, such as those treating diabetes or epilepsy, and optometrists, give advice more consistently than other groups dealing with less easily characterized risks, such as mental ill-health.[3]

- Doctors do not reliably ensure that appropriate information is provided to enable valid licensing decisions to be made (non-UK studies).[4]

- Lack of action by doctors to prevent driving by those with health-related impairment has led to severe accidents.[5]

- Drivers do not reliably follow advice from doctors (non-UK study).[6]

- It is not clear what role the following play in preventing valid advice on driving being given when appropriate during clinical consultations: lack of knowledge, lack of time, lack of feeling responsible, a concern not to cause friction with a patient.

- Health professionals in a number of jurisdictions have been considered liable, at least in part, when a driver seen by them as a patient has a health-related driving impairment but has not been warned of the risk and has then crashed and caused damage.[7]

Assessment of the need for advice

- Does the individual have a medical condition or impairment now which could affect driving safety?
  —If 'yes,' what is the right advice?
  —Can the individual realistically be expected to self-police their driving and modify or stop it if subjectively impaired?
  —Do I need to give the individual definite advice, eg to stop driving for a period?
  —If this is the recommendation, what determines when they can start driving

again? Time, lack of symptoms, cessation of medication, careful trial, eg emergency stopping when there may be post-operative pain-related limitations on pedal action?
  —Should the driver inform the DVLA or their insurer?
  —Should they stop driving permanently now?

- Could there be impairment in future? For example, the individual's visual problem or multiple sclerosis may progress and become more impairing. If so, the individual may need early guidance on work or where to live. Regular surveillance, or reporting any worsening, may be indicated.

- Does a young person or someone who may want a large vehicle (Group 2) licence have a condition which may limit their prospects of being licensed, eg poorly controlled epilepsy? If so, early vocational advice can help avoid future disappointments. However, if the condition is a static disability, such as movement limitation in a limb, you should avoid making assumptions about capability without recommending a practical assessment to review the scope for vehicle adaptation.

- Does the individual have work-related driving duties, whether in a car, using a large goods or passenger vehicle, or involving a special vehicle or an unusual driving environment (including working alone on a farm tractor)? Also do they drive any vehicles other than cars as part of leisure activities? This information may influence the advice you need to give.

- Is the individual already in contact with the licensing authority? If so, what is the current state of play and how can you best advise the individual until a decision on licensing has been reached?

- Has the individual lost their licence for health or alcohol/drugs-related reasons? If this is not a permanent ban, what steps do they have to take to regain their licence and can you assist?

- Does the individual hold any other licences (eg flying, seafaring, firearms) or undertake other activities where a medical condition could cause dangers to themselves or to others?
- Are you performing any procedure or giving any treatment that may impair driving temporarily or in the long term? What is the right advice to give prior to treatment, at consent and when treatment is completed?

- Can you choose an approach to treatment that will limit or avoid impairment of driving, such as a non-sedating therapy or keyhole surgery?

Giving advice

- People often forget advice that is given orally without reinforcement. Consider a definite dialogue on driving where your advice is repeated back to you by the

---

Clinical red flags for medically impaired driving[8]

If found in the course of a clinical consultation, the following symptoms, conditions and treatments should flag up the need to consider a patient's fitness to drive. In addition you will need to consider how best they can return to driving following injury and prior to any surgical procedure.

Acute events
- acute myocardial infarction
- acute stroke or other traumatic brain injury
- syncope and vertigo
- seizure
- surgery (including minor procedures if anaesthetics or sedation are used or if there is pain, postoperative medication or impairment to vision or to movement)
- delirium from any cause

Chronic medical conditions
- disease affecting vision
- cardiovascular disease – especially with risk of syncope or sudden recurrence
- neurological disease
- mental health problem
- metabolic disease/diabetes
- musculoskeletal disease
- chronic renal failure
- respiratory disease
- sleep disorder

Conditions with unpredictable episodic events
- pre-syncope or syncope
- angina
- seizure
- transient ischaemic attack

- hypoglycaemia
- sleep attack or cataplexy

Medications
- anticholinergics
- anti-epileptics
- antidepressants
- anti-emetics
- antihistamines
- antihypertensives
- antiparkinsonians
- antipsychotics
- benzodiazepines and other sedatives/anxiolytics
- muscle relaxants
- narcotic analgesics
- stimulants

Review of systems and symptoms
- general – fatigue, weakness
- head/ENT – headache, head trauma, visual changes, vertigo
- respiratory – shortness of breath
- cardiac – chest pain, dyspnoea on exertion, palpitations, sudden loss of consciousness
- musculoskeletal – muscle weakness/pain, joint stiffness/pain, decreased range of movements
- neurological – loss of consciousness, feelings of faintness, seizures, weakness/paralysis, tremors, loss of sensation, numbness, tingling
- psychiatric – depression, anxiety, memory loss, confusion, psychosis, mania

Fitness to drive should also be considered if the patient or a family member expresses concern about their safety to drive. The reasons for concern should be explored: recent crash or ticket, getting lost, poor vision, forgetfulness, confusion.

---

patient and supported by an information sheet.

- Advise specifically on the risks of medication and on the driver's need to read the label and package insert, and to follow the recommendations given.

- Record your advice on driving in the patient's notes.

- On occasions a letter to the patient confirming your advice or a 'no driving prescription' may help to reinforce the advice.

- Where you consider that the DVLA needs to be informed of a condition, indicate this clearly to the patient and follow up to check that they have followed your recommendations (see p. 24). Remember that it is the patient's responsibility to act on your advice.

The conflict between confidentiality and disclosure of a disability to the DVLA has been addressed by the General Medical Council (GMC). The basis for their guidance is the doctor's duty to disclose to protect the patient or others.[9] This has been amplified in several GMC statements, which differ in detail but all identify a set of principles and a procedure to follow.[10–12] The agreed wording for this requirement forms part of the DVLA's *At a Glance Guide* and drivers can be referred to it there.[13]

The stages are:

1. Recognition that the DVLA and not the doctor is legally responsible for deciding if an individual is medically unfit to drive. The DVLA needs to know when a driving licence holder has a condition which may, now or in the future, affect their safety as a driver.

2. Advice that a doctor should give:
   —Make sure that the patient understands that their condition may impair their ability to drive. If a patient is incapable of understanding this advice, eg because of dementia, the doctor should inform the DVLA immediately.

   —Otherwise explain to the patient that they have a legal duty to inform the DVLA about their condition.

3. If the patient refuses to accept the diagnosis or the effect of the condition on their ability to drive, the doctor can suggest that the patient seeks a second opinion, and make appropriate arrangements for them to do so. Advise the patient not to drive until the second opinion has been obtained.

4. If the patient continues to drive when they are not fit to do so, you should make every reasonable effort to persuade them to stop. This may include telling their next of kin.

5. If you do not manage to persuade the patient to stop driving, or you are given or find evidence that a patient is continuing to drive contrary to your advice, you should disclose relevant medical information immediately, in confidence, to the medical adviser at the DVLA.

6. Before giving information to the DVLA you should, whenever possible, inform the patient of your decision to do so. Once the DVLA has been informed, you should also write to the patient to confirm that disclosure has been made.

Doctors are expected to know of these guidelines and to have followed them if there is any challenge – either from the patient about clinical confidentiality or from other parties, such as insurers or representatives of those injured, who are concerned about liability when an accident is being investigated or when a claim is subsequently made against a driver. Other health professionals should follow their own professional guidelines.

Giving a patient adverse advice on their fitness to drive can be fraught because of its implications for employment, mobility and self-esteem. It will take additional time to explain to the driver and discuss the risks and their responsibility to refrain from driving or notify the licensing authority. In essence there is an inherent conflict between the public health and safety responsibilities of any health professional and their role as an advocate of what is best for their patient. The existence of the DVLA as the decision-taking body enables those with clinical responsibilities to avoid being the final arbiter of whether their patients can drive. However, health professionals' attitudes may be biased by the far more common experience of contact with someone whose licence has been removed than by the rarer one of knowing an individual who has caused or been the victim of a crash associated with impaired health. For road safety, as in any other effective preventative system, success in reducing risk can make us more concerned about the constraints we have to impose to keep potentially unsafe drivers off the roads than about the potential risks from not having them in place.

There are particular difficulties for all health professionals in dealing with conditions such as severe mental ill-health or early dementia, where insight may be lacking. There are also often valid concerns for the welfare and functioning of an individual if they cease to drive, in particular how best to balance the risks of road accidents against the social benefits of mobility and the costs and dangers of excluding people from society by limiting it. These can be particularly important when the individual's re-integration with society forms part of the therapeutic process after a period of mental illness and either the medication used or a recurrence of the symptoms may adversely influence safe driving. Such concerns about patient care and welfare can, however, cease to carry much weight when legal processes are used to attribute blame for a serious road crash!

- Where *new or temporary impairment* is associated with a medical condition or its treatment and the driver may not be aware of its impairing potential, it is good medical or other professional practice to inform the driver of this. When you are advising them, be specific about the nature and duration of any cessation or limitation to driving.

- For *short-term conditions*, you as the health professional will be the prime source of rational advice, as the licensing authority will not become involved.

- Even if the patient's condition is one where notification is indicated, there will be a period of weeks before a medical licensing decision is taken. During this period the decision on fitness to drive rests with the driver.

- However, it is the driver's responsibility to follow any professional advice on impairment, but unless the advice has been recorded the health professional is liable to challenge.

- The driver should be made aware that their insurance is almost certainly only valid if they are legally licensed to drive (see p. 29). Failure to disclose an impairing medical condition to the DVLA or driving while unfit to do so will be a breach of their insurance contract and so they will not be covered in the event of any crash, and especially one relating to their medical condition.

Oral advice given directly to the patient can be supplemented by the following.

- *Leaflets* provided in waiting areas for all patients to give general information and advice on impairment and driving. A number of the leading medical charities concerned with conditions that may have implications for driving, such as diabetes and dementia, produce useful material.

- *IT-based information systems* accessible by patients can be a source of more detailed advice on the consequences of individual conditions and treatments. The websites of a number of the leading medical charities provide good guidance (see Chapters 10–21).

- The use of *condition-specific leaflets* or personally printed proforma information during a consultation can be effective, especially if the recipient is then asked to rehearse the advice given or the leaflet re-iterates the advice given orally. This is common practice in some clinics where a limited range of diseases and forms of impairment is encountered. Later chapters of this book recommend the information to be given for some of the more common conditions that affect driving.

- The DVLA's *At A Glance Guide* to medical standards is the definitive statement on which medical licensing decisions are based. Its target audience is health professionals, but it is accessible to all and can be a useful way of explaining obligations and the likely outcome of declaring a condition to the DVLA. Printing off the relevant page may be a useful prompt to any patient who has been advised to notify the DVLA of a condition listed therein.[14] This will be particularly important if the patient has memory or recall problems.

When treatment is planned as a result of a consultation, it is important to ensure that the patient is aware of the implications for driving, just as they need to know about the anticipated duration and severity of any other limitations to their home or working life. At its simplest this will relate to the immediate aftermath of the treatment in terms of residual impairment from sedation and discomfort. Clear advice on whether it will be safe to drive home after any minor procedure is essential. Longer-term concerns include ensuring that pain or stiffness does not impair emergency procedures like sudden braking, or rearward vision. You should also ensure that the patient is aware of the time they may require to develop the skills needed to adapt to any personal limitations or to vehicle modifications, especially those affecting vision, cognition or musculoskeletal functions.

Many procedures, such as those that improve vision, prevent sleep apnoea or reduce the risk of a cardiac arrhythmia, will have benefits for driving safety and can enable those who have had their licences revoked to regain them. Prior to such procedures patients should be made

aware of the criteria for regaining their licence, both in terms of the duration of any period for recovery or adaptation to the results of the treatment and any specific performance standards that have to be met. Details are given in the DVLA's *At A Glance Guide*.

There are no specific standards for fitness to drive for a wide range of the less common medical conditions. You may need to develop your advice from first principles in such situations. Analogy with criteria for conditions listed by the DVLA that have similar patterns of impairment is usually the best route to use to develop such advice. Where this is not possible, assessment of current function by reference to subjective experiences of driving and of ability to cope with activities of daily living involving eye–brain–muscle coordination should be used. This needs to be supplemented with an estimate of the likelihood of sudden incapacity. Prognosis will determine how frequently you need to review the individual's capabilities. You need to note and may need to point out to patients that the legal basis for licence holding is not just the absence of any prescribed medical condition but also the absence of 'any other disability likely to cause the driving of a vehicle to be a source of danger to the public'. 'Likely' has been defined in legal judgments as 'more than a bare possibility but less than a probability'.

When giving travel advice it may be useful for you to discuss driving.

- A patient who has limited function but is still licensed to drive on British roads can find the different driving conditions in other countries, often coupled with use of an unfamiliar hire car on busy roads from an airport, difficult to cope with, and they may need to be advised to think hard before planning to do so.
- Road crashes are one of the most common causes of fatalities and serious injuries whilst travelling. Care is needed with all forms of vehicle use and when on the streets.

- Use of vehicles such as motorcycles and mopeds on poorly maintained roads, especially where crash helmets are not provided, has a high fatality rate.
- Long-haul flying can lead to impairment from sleep loss and from lack of adaptation to different time zones. Driving, particularly for long distances, after such flights is best postponed until after a period of rest.

Medical examiner function

DVLA requests

Health professionals may be asked to act as medical examiners to provide information or an appraisal about fitness to drive, usually for the DVLA but sometimes for an employer or as part of legal proceedings. A medical report will only be requested by the DVLA on a car driver if that driver declares a health problem when they first apply for a licence or subsequently. Often, information will also be obtained from the driver. Normally a questionnaire is sent asking for specific items of information, which the DVLA can use for their assessment, rather than seeking a clinical opinion. An exception to this is the position with insulin-using diabetics who drive vehicles in category C1 (3.5–7.5 tonne trucks), where a clinical opinion on the adequacy of their diabetic control and its stability is provided by a specialist diabetologist.

The health professional who provides any reports to the DVLA is acting as an expert source of information for the DVLA, whose aim is to ensure safety on the roads, and does not act as an advocate for the patient. The DVLA will enclose consent for disclosure from the licence holder. The speed with which the DVLA can give a decision to a driver is often determined by the time taken for return of such questionnaires by doctors, and your patient will benefit from a speedy response. There is a statutory obligation to 'defray any fees or other reasonable expenses of a registered medical practitioner' when providing a report on fitness to drive at the request of the DVLA (Road Traffic Act 1988 Section 94 [9]).

Group 2 driver medicals

Group 2 drivers (trucks and buses) need to provide the results of a medical examination on form D4[15] on application, at age 45 and periodically thereafter. When examining a driver and completing this form you are acting as a medical examiner on behalf of the DVLA in order to help minimize the accident risks from a large vehicle, even though the driver is responsible for payment.

For employment purposes

Should you be asked to advise on fitness to drive for employment purposes, you need to be very clear what is being requested, how the information will be used, and that the driver has been truly informed about the purposes of the examination and its consequences before giving their consent. If you are in any doubt you should recommend that the employer uses someone with competence in occupational medicine. They will be familiar with aspects such as confidentiality in the workplace setting, legal aspects of the contract of employment and any special job-related performance requirements. You may wish to indicate that, given consent, you will be ready to provide relevant clinical information to them.

Summary
- Advice on fitness to drive should form an integral part of many consultations.
- The health professional is the sole source of definitive advice on fitness to drive pending a DVLA decision.
- Advice on driving can be contentious and it may need reinforcement. If a patient does not comply with your advice, as a health professional you may need to notify the DVLA in the interests of public safety.
- When acting as a medical examiner for a third party, the health professional has a duty to give a true and fair view on a medical condition and its risks.

References

1. Information supplied by the Road Safety Statistics Branch, DfT.

2. Rabbitt P, *et al*. *Age, Health and Driving*. Basingstoke: AA Foundation for Road Safety Research, 2002.

3. Elwood P. Driving, mental illness and the role of the psychiatrist. *Ir J Psychol Med* 1998; **15**: 49–51.

4. Steier TS, *et al*. Are medical reports on fitness to drive trustworthy? *Postgrad Med J* 2003; **79**: 52–54.

5. *Medical Oversight of Non-Commercial Drivers*. Report NTSB/SIR-04/01. Highway Special Investigation. Washington DC: National Transportation Safety Board. www.ntsb.gov/publictn/2004/SIR0401.pdf

6. Maas R, Ventura, Kretzschmar C, *et al*. Syncope, driving recommendations, and clinical reality: survey of patients. *BMJ* 2003; **326**: 21.

7. Johnston C. Failure to report drivers' medical problems could have serious legal consequences for MDs. *Can Med Assoc J* 1993; **149**: 322–325.

8. *Physician's Guide to Assessing and Counseling Older Drivers*. Washington, DC: National Highway Transportation Safety Administration, Chapter 2: 4–7. www.nhtsa.dot.gov/people/injury/olddrive/ OlderDriversBook/pages/Chapter2.html

9. General Medical Council. Disclosure to Protect the Patient or Others. Para 27. Confidentiality: Protecting and Providing Information (April 2004). www.gmc-uk.org/guidance/library/confidentiality.asp

10. ibid: Question (FAQ) 17.

11. Driving the message home. *GMC News* 2001; **October**: 7.

12. Confidentiality: Protecting and Providing Information. Appendix 2 (with associated FAQs). London: General Medical Council, 2000.

13. *At A Glance Guide*. Swansea: DVLA. www.dvla.gov.uk/at_a_glance/what_is.htm

14. *At A Glance Guide*. Swansea: DVLA. www.dvla.gov.uk/at_a_glance/content.htm

15. www.direct.gov.uk/Diol1/DoItOnline/MotoringCategory/ fs/en?CONTENT_ID=10031645&chk=Mebj6X

5. Age, disability and assessment of needs for mobility

Age and driving performance
Advice on driving and mobility
Vehicle adaptation
Vehicle purchase for those with disabilities
Alternatives to car driving

Age and driving performance

Society implicitly tolerates some differences in the level of risk for and from different road users. This is within a framework of road safety which aims at overall reductions in harm while paying special attention to improving safety in high-risk groups. Examples of tolerated differences include:

- The increased level of risk in *new drivers* who, even after passing the driving test, need experience to learn all the required skills and attitudes for safe driving.

- Acceptance of some small increases in risk in *older drivers* in return for the benefits to the driver and to society of maintaining mobility.

- Degree of latitude society gives to drivers in terms of *choice of vehicle and driving style*.

The group of drivers with the highest crash risk is young males during the first few years after they have passed the driving test. It is notable that male drivers aged 17–20, and to a lesser extent females, have a far higher proportion of evening accidents than other drivers and that these peaks are highest between Friday and Sunday (Figure 5.1).

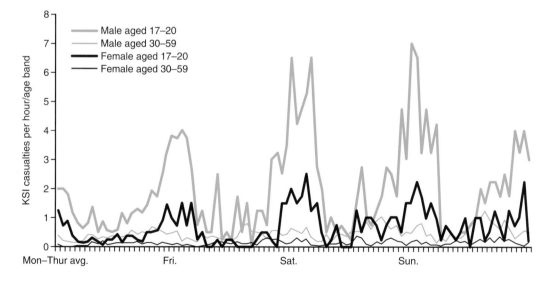

Figure 5.1
Average number of killed and seriously injured casualities in single vehicle accidents per hour, by day of week and age band, 2004.[1]

- Female drivers in all age groups have a lower rate than males.
- Disabled drivers with modified vehicles have an average risk.
- Drivers over the age of 70 show a small excess but this far lower than that of recently qualified drivers.
- The killed and seriously injured crash rate for motorcyclists is well in excess of that for car drivers.
- For some groups, such as motorcyclists and older drivers, a relatively high proportion of casualties occurs among the driver or rider.
- In others, such as young drivers and drivers of large goods vehicles, a higher proportion of casualties occurs among other road users.

Risk in older drivers

The increase in risk with age, even when the lower mileages driven by retired people is considered, is trivial compared with the risk in the young and inexperienced (Figure 5.2). The pattern also differs:[3]

- A fatal outcome in the older driver and passengers is more common, probably because of frailty or limited physiological reserve
- Elderly drivers rarely cause death or serious accident to other road users
- Minor vehicle damage represents the main increase in risk
- The attitude of other drivers to risk aversion or indecision in an elderly driver is often stated to be a cause of consequential risk but this is unproven.

Evidence – the older driver

- There is an extensive literature about driving performance in older drivers and about its association with other facets of ageing.[4]
- Older drivers are, in general, competent and responsible in monitoring and, if necessary, restricting their driving.
- Health, and in particular recent changes in health, is a major determinant of changes in driving patterns among older drivers.

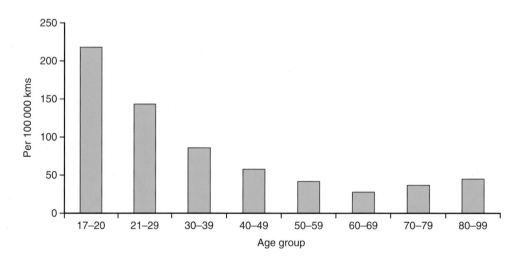

Figure 5.2
Driver/rider killed or seriously injured per 100 000 km travelled, 2004.[2]

- Older drivers hold stable opinions about mobility issues, valuing independence, but recognizing the need for advice when appropriate.

- The interactions between the processes of ageing, illness and the use of medication have been reviewed, indicating that a 'combined effects' risk analysis is required and noting that health professionals have a major part to play in this.[5]

- Increased age, even in the absence of any identifiable cause of disability, is associated with less effective visual function, slowing of cognitive processes and of the executive functions of the brain, as well as with reductions in strength and flexibility of musculoskeletal function.

- The way in which a driver's licence is applied for has been shown to have an effect. In those US states where drivers had to make applications in person, the over 85s had a lower driver fatality rate compared to middle-aged drivers in the same state.[6]

Most driver licensing systems use age as a criterion for increased frequency of re-licensing. Licensing decisions generally only relate to specified medical conditions but clinicians, in giving advice, will also need to consider:

- complex interactions among illness, medication and ageing processes

- sensory decrements, such as greater glare sensitivity or slower response to changed illumination

- slowing of cognitive processes, in particular specific limitations in ability to divide and prioritize attention

- the driver's own insight into their current capabilities

- weakness, tremor and pain limitation in motor functions, in particular the ability to turn the head when reversing

- any compensation by long experience, risk aversion and driving within known limitations.

Most decisions about adjusting driving patterns and continuing to drive when elderly are based on personal insight and self-policing. Both of these may be set aside for pressing social reasons, such as the need to transport a disabled partner. Drivers themselves, family members and clinicians are, in that order, the origin of decisions on ceasing to drive. Often this is as a consequence of an accident.

The clinician has an enabling role when there are no contraindications to driving. They can advise on the benefits of continuing mobility from driving and the ways in which this can be enhanced by vehicle choice or modification. They may also have formed their own view on the individual's unsuitability or, where insight is lacking, have been involved by relatives. Sometimes, especially where there is a dementing condition, the licensing authority may need to be informed in the absence of driver consent (see p. 36).

Mobility and driving can usefully form the basis of dialogue with an elderly patient before problems arise, as the social consequences, such as where to live and the use of public transport and taxis, can then be seen as a matter of rational choice rather than a closing down of opportunities.[7]

Advice on driving and mobility

In society, encouragement of safe driving and maintaining the benefits of mobility have relevance that is much wider than concerns about medical conditions and their effects on driving. However, a medical condition that impairs driving can cause major problems for an individual by removing the privilege of holding a driving licence, something which is only otherwise withdrawn for criminal behaviour.

The needs of certain groups of drivers may come to the attention of a health professional even when there is no specific medical condition that requires advice about driving. This may be because of either the importance of maintaining mobility or ensuring that driving is safe. Such advice is commonly needed:

- in those with new or established physical disabilities
- during pregnancy
- those with problems that make it difficult to get in or out of a vehicle
- when limited walking ability means that getting from vehicle to final destination is a problem
- where use of required safety aids such as seat belts or airbags is uncomfortable or risky
- most commonly, to take account of the effects of age on physical and mental capabilities.

Visual deterioration (see Chapter 8) and cognitive impairment (see Chapter 10), where the effects of ageing can sometimes but not always present as clinical problems, are discussed separately.

The best advice will depend on an assessment of the individual's situation. Sometimes this will simply be a direct response to a request for help, but for others a more detailed clinic- or vehicle-based evaluation will be needed. If vehicle modification is needed this should be based on a non-commercially-led assessment.

Clinic-based advice

Health professionals may need to give advice in anticipation of a question arising or in response to it.

- *Pregnancy*. The effects of change of shape on driving position need to be considered as well as the discomfort from prolonged journeys. There is inconclusive evidence of increased crash risks during pregnancy but not at a level or with sufficient validity to justify any restriction. It is prudent for the pregnant woman to respond to any self-awareness of the effects of tiredness, current mental state or discomfort, and to modify journey patterns. Occasionally specific advice may be needed, eg when short-term insulin is given during pregnancy.

- *Discomfort from wearing a seat belt*. Initially your advice should focus on posture, clothing and treatment of the underlying problem, as seat belts greatly reduce the serious injury risk after a collision. It may be possible to modify the seat belt, and details of suppliers of modifications are available via the Department for Transport's Mobility Advice and Information Service[8] or from other mobility centres (see p. 47). If these measures are not sufficient, eg for those with stomas or painful lesions on their chest or abdomen, there are arrangements for medical practitioners to grant exemption by issuing a form which the driver must carry.[9] (Blank medical exemption certificates, called 'Certificates of Exemption from Compulsory Seat Belt Wearing', are available to doctors only from the NHS distribution system. Tel: 0870 155 5455.)

- *Short stature leading to a driving position close to the wheel*. An airbag deploying after a collision may cause injury where its full expansion is constrained by a driver seated close to the wheel. Ideally a driver should be a minimum of 250 mm from the steering wheel in order to avoid any increased risk of injury from airbag deployment. Disarming the bag may very occasionally be justified, but alteration of the driving position, with modifications such as extensions to the foot pedals, may be appropriate. Great care is needed if the driving position is altered using cushions, as the driver may be in an unstable position and at greater risk of injury in the event of a crash.

- Some *physical limitations in drivers* may be amenable to modification by drivers themselves based on your advice. For example, a degree of pain-free neck and shoulder movement is needed for rear vision, especially when parking. A wide range of additional wide-angle and other mirrors is easily available and can reduce the need for neck movement. Drivers may be advised to experiment with various options and practise with them to decide for themselves what aid is most effective, taking care to avoid creating any new blind spots or other risks from the changes made.

- *Choice of car* can make a big difference to ease of access, and manufacturers are increasingly paying attention to this. This is relevant for regular passengers as well as for drivers. It is sensible to suggest that easy access, both to the seats and to the load-carrying area, is considered at an early stage in any condition that is likely to lead to persistent or progressive limitations on strength and flexibility. Ease of access can then be considered as and when a car is replaced. Simple mechanical aids, such as rotating seat cushions for either driver or passenger, are available. These may, however, increase the risk of injury in the event of a crash.

- *Disabled parking badges* (the Blue Badge Scheme) provide a national system of parking concessions for disabled people, allowing them to use dedicated bays near to shops and other facilities. The badge also gives other concessions.[10,11] Those who may be eligible should be referred to their local authority for more detailed information. Local authorities should also be able to provide information on other local schemes for alternative forms of transport, such as Dial-a-Ride, voluntary schemes, etc.

- As people age and restrictions on mobility from vehicle use become more likely, they can to an extent anticipate and minimize many of the problems by considering in advance where to live in terms of easy access to essential facilities on foot or by public transport and closeness to relatives or other potential carers.

Clinic-based assessment

The majority of assessments will be made by questioning an individual about their driving, identifying any difficulties, such as glare or problems with complex junctions, and then advising them on measures to overcome them. However, you may need to raise less apparent difficulties, such as the increasing prominence of post-lunch sleepiness with advancing age, as their significance for driving safety may not have been recognized by the driver. Similarly, progressive reductions on the acuity of distance vision are not readily recognized and you may need to give advice on regular eye testing and the use of glasses for driving.

Loss of insight about cognitive decline is common and it is the pace of decline during the later years of life rather than its existence that is the variable. Here you, as the health professional, need to take account of the views of relatives and regular passengers, as well as your own impression and any admitted driving errors.

The US National Highway Traffic Safety Administration, in association with the American Medical Association, has produced a practical clinic-based assessment framework for the older driver. Its components are grounded in experimental evidence that associates poor test results in groups studied with poor driving performance but there is, as yet, no validation of the whole test protocol (see p. 153). In essence the protocol provides a view of the key determinants of vision, cognition and motor function that are essential for safe driving. If satisfactory levels of performance are not achieved, then referral for a more detailed evaluation is recommended. If they are met, then, by implication, the present state of the driver is compatible with safe driving, from the functional point of view.

Car and driving assessments

Informal assessments of driving competence are, in practice, made by regular passengers in a car. Also, there may be evidence of recurrent minor vehicle damage, traffic violations and crashes. These assessments tend to be unstructured, but a simple list of prompts can be suggested to those concerned with the driving of relatives or friends. The questions reflect some of the common errors and aid a more structured discussion of any problems.

- Vision:
  - —Is the driver seeing static objects such as signs correctly?
  - —Are they detecting moving objects, especially at the periphery of vision, and following them with their eyes as needed?
  - —Does their driving suddenly become erratic after approaching headlamps or when driving into a low sun?

- Cognition:
  - —Does the driver judge approach speeds to junctions correctly?
  - —Do they judge the speed of other vehicles correctly, eg when turning or overtaking?
  - —Are they cautious when they approach a blind bend or junction, or when the behaviour of other road users, such as horses or children, is uncertain?
  - —In complex driving situations, such as at roundabouts, do they prioritize their actions sensibly, taking account of other road users and the intended direction of travel?
  - —Do they repeatedly get lost?
  - —Does their driving performance deteriorate because of fatigue and inattention, after a short period of driving?
  - —Do they show new or more severe levels of impulsiveness, aggression, anger, frustration or unjustified hesitation when driving?
  - —Are they aware of any personal limitations and do they adapt their driving style and pattern of car use to take account of these?

- Cognition and car control:
  - —Does the driver maintain a constant position in a lane?
  - —Do they keep a steady and sensible distance behind the vehicle in front?
  - —Do they correctly select and use gears? In particular, is third gear repeatedly selected for starting?
  - —Do they safely execute exits from side roads into a stream of traffic?
  - —Do they locate pedals reliably and use them in a coordinated way?
  - —Have their slow-speed manoeuvres, such as parking, passing through narrow gaps and moving in congested traffic, deteriorated?
  - —What are the circumstances in which any damage to car bodywork has arisen?

These pointers can serve as a guide to anyone who has raised concerns, and indicate a need for more detailed assessment or advice on limitation or cessation of driving. There are also a number of simple questionnaires that can be used to prompt discussion about driving performance (see Appendix 1). It is important to realize that the statutory driving test is only designed to examine competence and safety in a new driver. Most experienced drivers have developed an over-learned, hence persistent, and intuitive approach to driving which would not meet test requirements but which will normally be safe. The purpose of any assessment to look for subsequent impairment is simply to check that, whatever the details of the driving style, the sort of unsafe acts associated with sensory, cognitive or motor function in driving are not regularly occurring. Independent practical driving assessments are carried out by a variety of bodies. Local authority road safety officers and mobility centres are the most common, although the Institute of Advanced Motorists and some driving schools, such as the British School of Motoring, are also beginning to set up schemes, particularly for older drivers.

Road safety schemes

Some road safety units provide assessments of driving, either on request or periodically as a part of local road safety campaigns. These can give a more expert interpretation of capabilities. They are usually aimed at the older driver who does not have any particular physical limitations, who does not use or potentially need car modifications, and who is just starting to think about their future mobility.[12] Their orientation is practical and they do not look in any depth for subtle impairments of cognition, although these will be noted if they become apparent. The schemes vary from county to county, with some local authorities running education campaigns, providing literature-based information, while others provide a more practical in-car assessment service. The schemes offering practical assessment vary but generally involve approved driving instructors assessing the capabilities of older drivers in their own vehicles on the types of roads usually used by the individual driver. The outcomes of these assessments tend to fall into three categories:

- a satisfactory drive where a repeat assessment is recommended every three years, or sooner if there is a progressive medical condition
- an unsatisfactory drive which could be improved with a few driving lessons
- an unsafe drive, resulting in a recommendation for cessation of driving.

Information on schemes operating in your own area can be obtained from your local road safety officer, usually via the county council.

Mobility centres

In-depth assessment of driving, appropriate modifications to cars and training in their use are undertaken at centres run by the members of the Forum of Mobility Centres (www.mobility-centres.org.uk). There are 16 mobility centres in the UK, including one in Belfast. All have a central base where clients attend for the assessment. However, the Scottish centre undertakes assessments at a number of locations, and several other centres have recently set up satellite or outreach centres. These centres allow clients to access assessment services more easily. Some centres are within NHS trusts, others are charities or

Table 5.1
Medical conditions assessed at mobility centres, 2005 (Forum of Mobility Centres, www.mobility-centres.org.uk)

Neurological	60%
Physical	19%
Psychiatric	9%
Visual	4%
Other	8%

parts of charities and one is part of the Department for Transport. A wide range of conditions (Table 5.1) and ages of driver are seen but the main purpose of the assessment at a mobility centre is to provide independent advice that will enable an older or disabled individual to make an informed decision about their driving ability and the adaptations required to access a vehicle, stow equipment or operate the vehicle controls.

A special form of provisional driving licence can be issued by the DVLA to those who have had their licence revoked for medical reasons. This is issued to those who need to be assessed or to start re-learning to drive, often with a modified vehicle. As well as the instructors at mobility centres, there are approved instructors in most parts of the country who have special training in teaching people with disabilities to drive. The driving test is undertaken in the usual way at Driving Standards Agency test centres, with minor modifications as appropriate.

The duration of assessments varies depending on the functional needs of the individual but generally take between two and four hours. The components, depending on the reason for assessment, may include:

- vision screening and a health questionnaire, plus a review of any background information
- psychometric testing to assess facets such as processing of information, decision-taking and executive action, as well as the presence of dementia

- tests on a simple static rig to measure response times in a driving-related situation and to assess strength, stamina and flexibility of car control by arms and legs
- drive on private roads to assess car control, positioning in road and ability to follow instructions
- drive on public roads, generally using a dual-control car with one or two assessors. Some centres will, in certain circumstances, undertake the assessment in a client's own car. The drive normally follows a standard route for each centre and includes a variety of road and traffic conditions. The focus in this part of the assessment is to continue to assess car control, position at greater speed, attention, and the ability to deal with complex traffic situations. Tasks may be included in order to assess divided, selective and sustained attention, and to test memory. This test usually lasts between 40 and 60 minutes so that familiarity with the car is developed and signs of any rapid fall-off in performance can be seen.

Performance during all phases is recorded and progression to the on-road assessment is dependent on satisfactory performance in the centre and on its private roads. The Forum of Mobility Centres requires the mobility centres to work to minimum standards and is developing an educational programme to ensure staff conducting the assessments are competent to do so. Staff involved in assessment are a mix of approved driving instructors and healthcare professionals, occupational therapists being the most common health professionals involved. Some centres have input from clinical psychologists.

Assessment may be carried out at the individual's request, by referral from a health professional, Motability (see p. 49), solicitors, Access to Work, or, increasingly frequently, at the request of the DVLA. The information in Table 5.2 may provide useful reassurance that continuation of driving aided by helpful advice

is the most frequent result of an assessment. Except for assessments at the request of the DVLA, which are done to help determine whether or not to issue a licence and are at DVLA's expense, the individual being assessed normally pays. The results of assessments undertaken for the DVLA are communicated to the driver and to the DVLA. If the assessment is at the request of the individual or their adviser, the results are confidential to them and are not disclosed to others. They may be strongly advised to notify the DVLA, and this will be followed up with them. It is only rarely and when there are major safety risks, a lack of insight by the driver and a failure to notify despite several reminders, that the DVLA may be informed.

The report at the end of the assessment will indicate whether driving is safe, whether there are limitations that should be applied by the driver or whether driving should cease. Remedial training may be recommended and this can be undertaken either at the centre or by a specially trained driving instructor elsewhere. Vehicle choice and modifications may also be recommended. Any errors or lessons to be learned are explained to the driver at the end of the day. This process can be fraught if performance is poor and the driver is unaware of this or is in denial. However, all but the most impaired or unrealistic drivers

Table 5.2

Outcome of mobility centre assessments, 2005 (Forum of Mobility Centres, www.mobility-centres.org.uk).

Suitable to drive (with or without vehicle adaptations)	61%
Might be suitable (pre-learning assessment)	10%
Recommended for follow-up/training	13%
Advised against driving:	16%
• impaired perception	5%
• impaired decision-making/judgement	7%
• inadequate control/coordination	2%
• inadequate vision	2%
• medical problems, eg blackouts	0.4%

understand, if not welcome, having an assessor point out where dangerous situations were created or not avoided on the road test, and this is a powerful tool for persuasion. Nevertheless, the majority of those assessed are deemed fit, with or without some remedial training or car modifications.

Vehicle adaptation

Modification to a vehicle may be required to enable an individual to start driving or to continue after an illness or injury. Modifications can vary from the simple, such as additional mirrors or reshaped controls, to almost total rebuilds that, for example, allow an individual in a wheelchair to enter the vehicle and either to drive from their chair or to transfer from their chair to a driving position. Electronic links give flexibility in the position of controls and can allow the driver to use almost any level of strength and range of movement to control a vehicle. Such modifications are often individually tailored, can be very costly and require such major changes to the integrity of the vehicle that expert assessment and engineering is needed to effect them.

The mobility centres are able to give independent advice on the range of modifications that will enable an individual with a physical disability to return to driving. Some centres can also provide training in the use of such adaptations. Those requiring complex adaptations, such as electronic joystick operation of brake, accelerator and steering, may require assessment by the Department for Transport's own mobility centre, MAVIS, or by Motability. While many people have their adaptations fitted directly by the adaptation companies, a proper assessment of what is needed, free from commercial pressures, is desirable. A period of tuition using the new techniques is strongly recommended, as minor accidents can be common in the early stages of learning to use new controls.

Drivers of modified vehicles are issued with driving licences endorsed with codes that summarize the minimum solutions required to enable them to drive safely, and they are permitted to drive such vehicles only. The solutions noted in code form on the licence do not necessarily mean a physical adaptation to the vehicle. Rather, they mean that to drive the driver requires a method that is different from the standard method of using a manual car. For example, if someone is unable to move their right foot between the brake and accelerator, but is able to drive using their right foot to operate the accelerator and left foot to operate the brake, a licence code will be required even if there is no physical adaptation. Wherever possible, the adaptations are fitted in such a way that the standard vehicle controls can still be used. However, because of the structure of some of the adaptations, there may be an increased risk of injury in the event of an accident. In a few instances, where the adaptations are more complex, it is not possible for the standard car controls to be used, making the vehicle impossible or dangerous for another driver to drive. This can cause problems in the event of a breakdown or unexpected illness.

Modifications may also be needed to enable severely disabled passengers to travel as passengers, either seated in their wheelchair, or through modifications to make access easier, such as swivel seats and personal hoists. The mobility centres can provide advice on these.

Vehicle purchase for those with disabilities

The benefits of personal vehicle use for those with immobilizing disabilities or with an inability to use public transport are recognized. Motability (www.motability.co.uk) subsidizes schemes for car leasing, whether or not the vehicle needs adaptation.[13] Generally the disabled individual is responsible for paying for their own adaptations, although they can apply to Motability for grant aid towards the cost of these adaptations. There are clear eligibility criteria for the scheme.

Alternatives to car driving

Loss of the mobility provided by driving is life-changing. In older people it is commonly seen as one of the major downward steps of old age. Health professionals frequently become involved in advice about ceasing to drive and its consequences, usually when it becomes inevitable, but sometimes in advance when a planned series of steps can be taken to minimize its impact. The following are some of the key aspects:

- When feasible and planned, living within *walking distance* of essential amenities or near to regular and accessible public transport will ease the transition.

- Those who have been users of *public transport* earlier in life return to it in a better informed way than those who have always relied on cars. Advice on finding out about concessionary fares, timetables and any special services, such as Dial-a-Ride for those with special needs, is helpful.

- It may be helpful to indicate that the costs of owning and running a car are the same as about 2000 miles of taxi travel each year. *Taxi use* may be an economically sound alternative to driving, possibly supplemented by public transport for longer journeys.

- Where an individual's mobility is limited, they may consider the use of a *powered wheelchair or powered mobility scooter*. Prior to purchase, they or their carer will need to carefully consider issues such as transfer to and from the chair, ramp access to storage, battery recharging, the quality and dangers of pavement and road surfaces, and any barriers such as stairs on essential routes. The purchaser also needs to consider whether travel will be on crowded roads or pavements and how they will interact with other road and footway users. They will also need to make a sound estimate of use and to recognize associated problems such as coldness, breakdowns and maintenance requirements. Some chairs and scooters are sold in the home by means of

aggressive sales tactics; others may be purchased second hand without maintenance arrangements. A good and non-commercially motivated assessment of use, needs, options and costs is needed. Some of the mobility centres and some disability groups can supply this. Once such a vehicle is purchased, it is desirable for the driver to have training in use as well as insurance both of the item and against third-party risks, such as damage to property or injury to others. Arrangements also can be made for help in the event of a breakdown or other mishap while it is being used.

- The Disabled Persons' Advisory Committee (DPTAC; www.dptac.gov.uk) produces a range of useful publications and links to other sources of advice.

Summary

- Crash risks are highest in new, young, male drivers. There is a small increase late in life.
- Driving brings mobility benefits that are particularly important for those with disabilities and for older people.
- Assessment of factors likely to impair driving performance can be done in a number of ways. It provides the basis for advising on whether driving can continue and on the means that can be used to remain driving safely.
- Vehicles may be adapted to meet the needs of many drivers with disabilities.
- If driving is likely to cease, then good planning and advice can help to minimize the adverse effects.

References

1. Department for Transport. *Road Safety Statistics (SR5)*. London: The Stationery Office.

2. Ibid.

3. *Older Drivers: A Literature Review*. Road Safety Research Report No 25. London: Department for Transport, 2001. www.dft.gov.uk/stellent/groups/dft_rdsafety/documents/page/dft_rdsafety_504602.hcsp

4. Rabbitt P, *et al. Age, Health and Driving*. Basingstoke: AA Foundation for Road Safety Research, 2002.

5. Holland C, Handley S, Feetam C. *Older Drivers, Illness and Medication*. Research Report 39. London: Department for Transport, 2003. www.dft.gov.uk/stellent/groups/dft_rdsafety/documents/divisionhomepage/030261.hcsp

6. Grabowski DC, Campbell CM, Morrisey MA. Elderly licensure laws and motor vehicle fatalities. *JAMA* 2004; **291**: 2840–2846.

7. *Drive On! Advice for Older Drivers*. London: Department for Transport 2002, THINK! campaign leaflet T/INF/263. www.thinkroadsafety.gov.uk/advice/pdf/olderdrivers01.pdf

8. www.dft.gov.uk/stellent/groups/dft_mobility/documents/page/dft_mobility_503255.hcsp

9. *Medical Exemption from Compulsory Seat Belt Wearing:* *Guidance for Medical Practitioners*. London: Department for Environment, Transport and the Regions, 1999. (Available from Department for Transport.)

10. www.dft.gov.uk/access

11. www.direct.gov.uk/DisabledPeople/MotoringAnd Transport/MotoringAndTransportArticles/fs/en?CONTENT_ ID=4001061&chk=lH4OUe

12. Barham P, Oxley P, Taylor N, Roberts S. Review of Driving Advice/Assessment Services for Older Drivers Throughout the UK. Unpublished report commissioned by Department for Transport, 2005.

13. *Get Motoring. Finding and Financing Your Car – A Practical Guide for the Disabled Motorist*. London: RADAR, 2005. www.radar.org.uk/radarwebsite/RadarFiles/Documents/ Get%20Motoring.pdf

conditions, eg epilepsy or cardiac arrhythmia. There is sound evidence that some conditions that cause sudden changes to driving performance, eg sleep apnoea, seizures and hypoglycaemic episodes in insulin users, are a cause of crashes.

Estimates of the risks from such episodic incapacity can only be based on studies of populations who have the medical condition. As a consequence they cannot provide the basis for making an assessment of risk specific to an individual, except to a limited extent when risk levels within a population with a particular diagnosis can be stratified, eg by the time since the last incapacitating event, so that it is possible to estimate the risk for those individuals who lie within a particular stratum. This sort of evidence is not available from crash data unless there are reliable population reference statistics.

Information on the links between severity of the condition and frequency of incapacitation has to be derived from clinical studies of disease natural history. This may be done by reference to predictive screening tests, such as the Bruce protocol exercise ECG in those with ischaemic heart disease, or by reference to studies that show that certain prognostic indicators, eg length of time since last seizure, are valid indicators of the future probability of another event.

For episodic impairments it should, in principle, be possible to determine the frequency of incapacitating episodes. However, as much of the available data relate to clinical endpoints such as hospital admissions or deaths rather than to the rapid onset of disabling episodes that are likely to cause a road crash, it is difficult to extrapolate from clinical event rates to driving risks.

- *The speed of onset of an episode of impairment can be critical.* Where, as with major seizures, the onset is very rapid, and hence remedial action is unlikely, the incidence of episodes can reasonably be used to predict, or at least to stratify, the risk of loss of control of a vehicle and

hence a crash, using incidence data from the wider population of those liable to seizures. However, if the onset is slower, as in the case of most cardiac events, where incapacitation is from cerebral ischaemia, usually arising several tens of seconds after other symptoms of the cardiac event, there is scope for taking remedial action. In such cases clinically based evidence on the frequency of rapid incapacitation may overestimate driving risk. The most common pattern in cardiac death at the wheel is not a crash but a vehicle pulled into the side of the road, often with the engine turned off and the handbrake applied. An increased risk of sudden incapacitation can sometimes be predicted in the absence of a prior event, eg seizures after a head injury, intracranial surgery, a cerebral metastasis secondary to a lung cancer, or the discharge of an implanted cardiac defibrillator.

- *Behavioural factors* play a major part in determining whether the driver takes immediate action to cease driving when they first perceive acutely impairing symptoms. A driver who is on the verge of sleep may pull in, but bad judgement arising from the very fatigue that is leading to sleep may mean that they do not break the journey. Some drivers using insulin are much more meticulous than others in ensuring that they avoid hypoglycaemia or carry a source of glucose and eat it. The early effects of hypoglycaemia can themselves adversely influence behaviour by disinhibiting anger or impetuousness or by clouding awareness of the need to stop and take glucose. In such circumstances the need to avoid crashes in those with behaviour patterns which pose a risk can mean that other insulin-using drivers are restricted too. This precautionary approach is needed unless it is possible to identify those in high and low behavioural risk groups effectively and efficiently and it is then administratively practicable to apply different standards to each.

Prognosis

For most episodes of ill-health and injury there is a return to normal function. Limitations on driving are needed when there is acute impairment and these are applied by the driver either on their own initiative or on the advice of a health professional. However, such limitations cease to be relevant and are informally dropped on recovery when any impairing effects have gone.

An illness or injury may leave the individual with residual disability, either from a constantly impaired state of functioning, such as a fixed joint, or with an increased likelihood of sudden incapacitation, such as insulin-treated type 1 diabetes.

Many chronic diseases have a progressive course, leading either to increasing impairment, as in motor neurone disease, or to episodes or exacerbations where function declines with each event.

For some conditions the pattern of future impairment is complex.

- *Multiple sclerosis* will show a pattern of remission and progression. During remissions the risks of errors or loss of vehicle control will be low, but during exacerbations sensory, cognitive or motor impairment may increase the likelihood of errors or loss of car control. Other effects of the condition such as fatigue may show a much more variable pattern day by day.

- A range of *mental health conditions* similarly have a prognosis comprising periods of remission and exacerbation, where often the crash risk varies markedly. For example, in bipolar disorders there is impulsiveness and lack of insight at the onset of manic phases.

- *Alcohol and substance misuse* can show similar periods of abstinence and misuse with very different levels of risk, both from the acutely impairing effects of the substance and from progressive impairments from secondary illnesses.

- After a *stroke* caused by atheromatous arterial disease there may be a range of sensory, cognitive and motor impairments and a variable pace of recovery. Some impairments will be apparent to the individual but others, such as cognitive loss, inattention to one side or loss of visual field may not. Because of the underlying disease process, the individual will have an increased risk of both further strokes and related arterial conditions, such as myocardial infarction.

- For many conditions such as the *recurrence of a cancer*, unless it presents with a seizure from a cerebral secondary, changes are not on a timescale where driving performance will suddenly worsen, although effects such as fatigue, progressive muscular weakness or the use of strong analgesics that will adversely affect driving can be anticipated.

- *Pain* from any cause may be impairing. This may be as a result of associated fatigue or, where pain is musculoskeletal, the movements such as use of pedals or head turning which are needed for safe driving may be inhibited either by actual pain or by guarding behaviour to avoid provocation.

Risk analysis

Given the complex pattern of impairment that can affect safe driving, the scope for developing a single quantitative measure of crash risk attributable to health-related impairment is severely limited.

- Within the range of severities for a single condition or for related conditions with common forms of impairment, it will sometimes be possible to *stratify the risk for different identifiable sub-groups*. Examples include the use of time since last seizure in those at risk of recurrence, or the use of the Bruce protocol exercise ECG to evaluate the probability of a future incapacitating cardiac event.

- Where the condition is stable, the use of *simulation or structured test drives* may provide information that enables an individual to be ranked in relation to others in terms of risk of driver error or loss of car control.

In part because of these limitations, many of the criteria used for licensing decisions are based in large measure on specialist consensus rather than rigorous risk assessment. This is particularly so in areas such as psychiatric disorders, where any evidence of risk specific to driving reflects many uncertainties and has to be seen as part of a larger picture of the condition and its treatment.

Where there are quantitative data, eg on risks of seizure or cardiac event, the application of quantitative methods of risk assessment may be useful. However, very few studies have sufficient precision and so quantitative estimates of risk have confidence intervals that are so large as to make the results of very limited use.[1–3] It is however often possible to stratify risk among groups who have similar conditions, a good example being the use of the Bruce protocol exercise ECG as a predictor of recurrence in a wide range of arterial conditions.[4,5]

Tolerability of excess risk

Decisions on medical conditions and fitness to drive have been taken for some 70 years. Because of this there is not a blank slate for decisions on risk assessment and tolerability. Certain principles and licensing controls on a range of medical conditions are specified in European Union directives and are codified in UK law (see p. 21 and p. 28). This means that current decisions about setting and changing medical fitness criteria are about modification and not about how they can be created from scratch. As a result there have been few instances where political processes have been fully used to review evidence of risk and to make judgements on behalf of society about how much excess risk is acceptable.

In practice pragmatic decisions have been taken and then their scope extended as the limited available evidence on crash risk has indicated that they were justified. A good example is the use of a <2% per annum risk of seizure for Group 2 vehicle driving and a <20% risk for Group 1. This was initially applied to those with a history of head injury and then extended to all those with an excess risk of seizure. It is now being used as an informal benchmark for other forms of sudden incapacitation. This has enabled some drivers to return to driving who would have had their licences permanently removed when there were absolute prohibitions on those with a history of repeated seizures. Measurement of the validity of such an approach to risk reduction is not easy, but there have been very few reported crashes attributable to seizure in those on whom decisions have been taken based on these criteria. However, crashes continue to occur in those drivers who have not complied with the requirement to notify the licensing authority.

The levels of excess crash risk associated with both youth and old age, as well as inexperience and the level of blood alcohol at which a driver can be prosecuted, have in effect created some benchmark levels which could be applied to health-related forms of impairment. But very different attitudes are taken in these cases.

- Inevitably the *inexperienced driver* gains experience. As most people learn to drive in their late teens and early 20s, it is impossible to separate the effects of inexperience and youthful behaviour. Extrapolation using this group as a benchmark for the limits of acceptable risk is not supported. The high level of risk is seen more as a stimulus to improve driver training and to structure the experience gained in the first few years after passing the test in a better way.

- Both the elderly themselves and the rest of society gain huge benefits from *older people* remaining mobile and self-sufficient. Similarly the crash incidence for older drivers is not an acceptable benchmark for tolerable risk.

- The *alcohol limit* by no means indicates an acceptable level of risk but is a politically determined criterion for enforcement.

It is not seen as relevant to use comparisons with measured excesses of crash risk in these groups for determining the tolerability of crash risk from health-related impairment.

More generally, in the wake of disability legislation, there are assumptions that individuals will be assessed in terms of their personal capabilities and that they will not be categorized using group stereotypes about capability. This individual approach is the one already used in the assessment of drivers in mobility centres, both to specify vehicle modifications and to assess driving capability (see p. 47). Assessment is very much based on the experience of the assessors and the structure of the assessment. It is only applicable to stable or predictable forms of impairment.

Any decisions about an individual's risk of a recurrence of some episodic forms of impairment have to bring together population-based evaluations of prognosis and an assessment of the quality of an individual's control of their condition. Examples where this approach can be considered include the risk of hypoglycaemia from the use of insulin or the quality of sleep and wakefulness in treated sleep apnoea. Taken together, prognosis and an individual's ability to control their disease can sometimes form the basis for a judgement on personal fitness to drive. Objective information on the individual's quality of disease management may be collected and used in making judgements on individual fitness. For example, blood glucose levels may be recorded by meters that have a memory which logs the time of sampling and the results; modern continuous positive airway pressure (CPAP) machines used to treat sleep apnoea can record the times when they are in use.

Personal risk evaluations may be based on

medical data, such as exercise ECG testing, which have been shown to predict the probability of a future cardiac event. Here the strength of the method lies in its well established link with disease recurrence, while its weakness comes from the lack of evidence linking such recurrences to excess crash risk. As the individual tested will be aware of whether they have safely completed the test at the time and may be shown ECG evidence of ischaemic change on exercise, this method does have a higher face value for those assessed and found unfit than any simple categorization of fitness to drive by condition.

The greater consequential damage associated with large vehicles, especially those carrying passengers or dangerous goods, and the higher expectations of fare-paying passengers that drivers be unimpaired, make more stringent, and hence discriminatory, fitness standards justifiable for such licences (see p. 22). There is a well established but not clearly formulated set of public and political expectations that more stringent criteria for fitness are appropriate for drivers of large vehicles.

Vehicles used on worksites, including airports, farms, mines, docks and construction sites, may differ in their performance characteristics from those used on the roads. For example, a forklift truck driver often needs easily to turn their head as they navigate large loads around a warehouse. They may need additional selection and surveillance if it is a cold store. Hence, while road-driving standards may be used as a benchmark, the specific risks also need to be taken into account when deciding on an individual's suitability for a specific driving task. The scope for consequential damage on different worksites may also vary greatly. For example, multiple passenger casualties may be caused by a vehicle interfering with the safe landing of an aircraft. By contrast, there can be considerable excess personal risk, but no risk to others, when working alone on a farm tractor, often on unstable ground. The basis for judgements on tolerability of risk from health-related impairment on worksites may diverge from those used for the public highway, although the DVLA Group 1 and 2 standards are commonly used as benchmarks for worksite driving.

Summary

- The evidence base for fitness standards for driving is less than perfect but is being improved.

- Current standards have evolved and are based on a mix of evidence, expert opinion, consensus and experience in use.

- Medical licensing standards only cover long-term conditions, and much risk reduction depends on decisions about whether to drive and on the recommendations of health advisers.

- Different forms of impairment need to be assessed in different ways and there is a move towards individual assessment where feasible.

- At present there is no valid basis for setting a single quantitative limit on the acceptable level of excess risk in drivers from health-related impairment, but there is scope for stratifying risk among those with similar conditions.

References

1. Spencer M. *The Role of Risk Analysis in the Evaluation of Fitness to Drive*. Road Safety Research Report No. 40. London: Department for Transport, 2003. www.dft.gov.uk/stellent/groups/dft_rdsafety/documents/divisionhomepage/030264.hcsp

2. Spencer M. *Risk Analysis and Fitness to Drive: Evaluation of Sensitivity Issues*. Road Safety Research Report No. 41. London: Department for Transport, 2003. www.dft.gov.uk/stellent/groups/dft_rdsafety/documents/divisionhomepage/030264.hcsp

3. Spencer MB, Carter T, Nicholson AN. Limitations of risk analysis in the determination of medical factors in road vehicle accidents. *Clin Med* 2004; **4**: 50–53.

4. Weiner DA, Ryan TJ, McCabe CH, *et al.* Prognostic importance of a clinical profile and exercise test in medically treated patients with coronary artery disease. *J Am Coll Cardiol* 1984; **3**: 772–779.

5. McIntyre H. The ability to predict future cardiac events based on the exercise ECG in patients with known coronary artery disease. *Expert Consensus Workshop: Driving Safety and Cardiac Ischaemia*. London: Department for Transport, 2006.

7. Driving for work

Common work-related driving tasks
Work-related driving – general issues

Driving is an important part of many people's work. This may be on the public highway, within a work area or a mixture of both. It may involve very different sorts of vehicles from those used outside work, as well as driving in environments that differ markedly from public roads. Driving may be as:

- an employee, when the employer has certain responsibilities to ensure safe working conditions
- as a contractor, where the client may place conditions on the drivers used
- as a self-employed individual.

Evidence – work-related driving

- In Great Britain work-related driving is estimated to result in 25–33% of all fatal and serious accidents on public roads. This amounts to around 1000 road fatalities each year. It is far in excess of the number of fatal accidents arising within workplaces.[1]
- Forklift trucks cause 8000 (10 fatal) accidents per year. Common causes for this include poor visibility and lack of clearly demarcated and observed areas for vehicles and for pedestrians.[2]
- Vehicle roll-over because of unstable slopes and/or incorrect loading causes regular fatalities on farms and construction sites. The risk can be reduced by the use of roll-over indicators to identify when the vehicle is at risk from its inclination and roll-over

protection to reduce crush injuries if roll-over occurs.
- The diversity of conditions within workplaces means that general approaches to safe driving have to be complemented by site-specific risk assessments and accident mitigation measures.

Common work-related driving tasks

- *Car driving on public roads for work* other than commuting to and from the usual place of work (a tax-based definition). Examples are professional service providers, sales staff and managers of multisite businesses. Some drivers may have to handle heavy and awkward samples or equipment. The manual handling risks need to be considered and may be reduced by using vehicles such as estate cars which do not have a high sill at the rear. Normal car driving risks and fitness requirements apply, but drivers may be subject to time pressures, long working hours and the need to drive even when not feeling well. Company car drivers are estimated to have up to 50% more accidents than those driving for domestic purposes.[3]
- *Delivery driving*. This can be local or cover a regional area, with variable vehicle size and hence a range of licence requirements. In addition to the requirements for driving a car as part of work, delivery drivers need to be able to handle loads on and off a vehicle. An assessment of the task and of the design of the vehicle may be needed. They may encounter disrupted delivery schedules, and hence difficulty in maintaining a stable pattern of work and eating.
- *Trunk route driving*, including international journeys. This will usually be in a large vehicle, driving for long hours and possibly with a relief driver. Drivers may be away from home for long periods. They may be tempted to compromise on sleep and food requirements; they may also need to handle

unfamiliar traffic conditions and administrative demands.

- *Passenger transport – taxi, private hire and minibus.* Passengers have expectations of a safe driver and reliable service. Drivers will often need to be able to assist disabled passengers and stow disability aids and other luggage. They may experience threats from passengers. Taxis are licensed by local authorities, which are responsible for medical standards of fitness. The majority use the Group 2 standards, but may adopt a degree of discretion about individual cases.[4] Drivers need to meet the physical and mental demands of the task and comply with local licensing authority requirements on competence, conduct and fitness.

- *Passenger transport – bus and coach.* These are large vehicles (Group 2) with many passengers, and the consequential harm from a crash can include multiple casualties. Tasks vary from driving urban buses with short journeys on set routes and multiple pick-ups (with the bus repeatedly driven towards waiting passengers) to long-haul international coach-driving. The driver may also be acting as a guide or collecting fares. Drivers can be self-employed, contracted or employed by the operator. The driver needs to meet Group 2 medical standards as well as the competency and conduct requirements of their employer or the client for the contract. The driver also needs to have good communication skills.

- *Emergency services – fire, police, ambulance, coastguard.* Demands include fast driving in emergencies, with rapid decisions about taking advantage of other traffic giving way to blue lights and sirens. Emergency services have to perform demanding and often dangerous tasks at the site of the emergency. Drivers need to make extensive use of radio communications. Employers normally have their own fitness standards in addition to those required by the DVLA (fire appliances usually are Group 2 vehicles because of size). These standards may reflect fitness requirements for emergency duties, such as carrying, running, wearing protective apparatus, firearms use, as well as for driving under emergency conditions.

- *Worksite materials handling.* Extensive use is made of forklift trucks, etc. Where these are only used within a workplace and not on public roads, a DVLA licence is not a requirement. The job demands will vary, but commonly work is in congested areas where there are other workers and sometimes members of the public. The driver's vision may be obscured by loads, and flexibility may be needed to see to the rear during frequent reverse movements. Employers should have competence and fitness requirements based on a risk assessment of the task. These should be in accordance with Health and Safety Executive (HSE) or other relevant guidance. Vehicles may be used in unusual environments such as cold stores or places where there are risks from exposure to harmful agents such as dusts, hot items or corrosive substances. Criteria for fitness to drive should be based on a location-specific risk assessment. The DVLA medical standards are commonly used as benchmarks.

- *Construction site, quarry, mine and dock mobile plant.* This includes cranes, straddle carriers for containers, massive off-road trucks and digging equipment. Unstable slopes, unguarded edges and poor weather conditions are frequent. Assessments of the site and the risks from the types of plant used are the basis for protection. Competence and fitness standards form part of this. For some tasks, such as mobile crane use, a high level of skill in depth perception is needed. HSE and sector trade association guidance should form the basis for assessment.[5] The DVLA medical standards are commonly used as benchmarks.

- *Farm tractors, harvesters, all-terrain vehicles and forestry vehicles.* Lone working is common, with the driver sometimes having to handle awkward loads or work on unstable slopes. Dangerous materials may be used, such as pesticides. There may be associated risks of trauma or entrapment from farm implements, often driven from tractor power take-offs. Work areas may also be animal-holding places or even act as play areas for children on the farm. DVLA licensing is required only if the vehicle is used on public roads. Drivers are often self-employed, so precautions depend on personal training, competence and readiness to follow safe procedures. Some engineering protection is possible, eg anti-roll-over bars/cabs on tractors, guarded power take-offs and interlocks to prevent the activation of farm machinery during maintenance. The driver will need advice on the dangers in the event that they develop a medical condition with risk of driving impairment. It is unlikely that such drivers will have access to advice on their health and driving other than from the health professionals they see clinically, so it is important to give any patient with such work clear and valid advice.

- *Airside driving at airports.* A wide variety of specialist vehicles are used for fuelling, passenger handling, loading food and baggage on to aircraft, and for towing aircraft. The environment is visually complex and reliant on observation of strict driving protocols. Correct recognition of colour light signals in low light conditions and of port and starboard wingtip lights is essential. The major requirement is for a high level of competence and for reliable observance of rules. Medically the DVLA Group 2 standards are commonly used as a benchmark for fitness, with an additional requirement for normal colour vision.

Work-related driving – general issues

Fitness standards

On public roads DVLA standards represent minimum ones; employers and those who engage contractors can require additional ones. It is wise only to introduce additional criteria on the advice of someone with knowledge of the tasks and credentials in occupational medicine. One of the most straightforward approaches is to confirm full compliance with the relevant DVLA standards by strengthening the disclosure obligations of the licence holder by:

- monitoring absences to identify conditions that may impair driving
- a requirement to cease driving in the presence of specified medical conditions or types of medication use, with maintenance of employment
- periodic surveillance for common forms of impairment such as reduced visual acuity.

Frequently DVLA Group 2 standards are adopted for certain groups of driver, even when Group 1 standards are the legal requirement. Where this approach is adopted, it will often be desirable for employers, guided by a health adviser, to apply a measure of discretion, eg by allowing some drivers who do not meet these standards to continue to drive, either because the job or vehicle can be modified in some way to reduce risk or because a higher level of surveillance of health or performance can be put in place than is possible for the general public. The use of Group 2 medical standards can be seen as providing a higher standard of fitness. However, their use can cause problems.

- The DVLA requires and will pay for additional tests, such as a Bruce protocol ECG after a heart attack, in holders of full Group 2 licences. Any employer using the Group 2 medical standards as non-discretionary criteria rather than as a benchmark, with a degree of discretion based on their assessment of risk, needs to accept that such costs become their responsibility.
- An employee could challenge the use of these standards at an industrial tribunal if they were discriminated against or lost their job. There has been a test case on

this which was decided on appeal.[6] The employer (the Post Office) won, but only because they had a rationale for their policy (of not allowing insulin users to drive postal collection and delivery vans) based on their pattern of work in peopled areas, and because this policy was written in advance and not developed to deal with the specific case of the complainant.

Risk assessment

The employer has a responsibility to undertake a risk assessment under the Health and Safety at Work Act 1974 and regulations made under it. The duty applies to driving that forms a part of their employees' work, even when on public roads, although here it is the provisions of the Road Traffic Act 1988 that will usually form the initial basis for enforcement, with recourse to health and safety legislation when, for example, it is found that the driver has been having to drive for an excessive time or when impaired by a very long working day.

The aim of the assessment is to identify the risks from the work activity to that employee and to others, including the public, so that steps can be taken to reduce it. The assessment should address:

- risks to the driver while driving, whether from a crash or from back problems as a result of poorly designed seating and controls or because of manual handling when loading and unloading the vehicle
- risks to the public, including crash risk and, for example, the consequence of the driver shedding the load or losing containment of a hazardous substance
- working environment factors, such as temperature and instability, to assess the adequacy of safeguards in the working environment, such as segregation of vehicles lanes.

In all but the smallest workplaces the assessment needs to be written, although parts can be covered by reference to other guidance from the HSE, trade associations, etc.

Risk management

The approach to management of driving risks at work should be derived from the overall risk assessment. Of particular relevance to health professionals are:

- the application of fitness criteria over and above those of the DVLA
- policies on the use of medication while driving
- approaches to return to work as a driver after illness or injury.

The employer should have used suitable expertise in developing these approaches. This would normally be based on the advice of an occupational physician, although codified or recommended standards for some groups, such as emergency service drivers, have been developed by national bodies.

For taxi drivers, the House of Commons Select Committee report, *Taxi and Private Hire Vehicles*, recommended in 1995 that taxi licence applicants should pass a medical examination. The Medical Commission for Accident Prevention recommended in 1995 that Group 2 medical standards should be used because of the need to ensure that fare-paying passengers were not put at unnecessary risk. Its recommendation has been endorsed by various expert bodies subsequently. It is, however, contested at times, especially in relation to the risk of seizures and to diabetes that appears to be reliably managed on insulin.

Contract and self-employed drivers

Larger contractors may have their own in-company policies for drivers. Major users of contract and self-employed drivers, such as supermarkets and oil companies, may include in their contracts fitness and competency requirements over and above those of the DVLA. Recently this has been notable in relation to sleep and fatigue, not least to ensure that drivers do not undertake multiple contracts at the same time. Where smaller contractors or the self-employed are working for small clients, special fitness standards, risk assessment and risk management are usually less reliably in place. The health professional may need to give very firm advice if they consider that there is a risk from their patient driving, as there are likely to be strong economic incentives to continue.

Hours of work

For Group 2 drivers there are European Union-wide requirements for limits to driving hours and these are recorded by the tachograph, the records of which may be required as proof of compliance. Employers and owner-drivers have been prosecuted when these requirements have been breached and there have been accidents that could have been caused by fatigue. The hours driven are recorded but waiting time is not, and so the driver can have a long working day, eg with periods of hours waiting for a supermarket to accept a delivery, without the rules being broken but with effects on driver fatigue.

Many larger employers now accept that there are risks from prolonged driving at the end of the working day and are more positive about avoiding these by advising employees to stay overnight or to use public transport. Financial incentives to driving, such as generous mileage rates or more favourable tax treatment if a car is mainly used for company business, need to be seen as disincentives to good risk management.

The restrictions on working and driving hours are seen as benefiting safety by reducing fatigue and the risk of falling asleep (see Chapter 21). Their originators also see them as a means to improve the work–life balance and to ensure that forcing people to work long hours is not a means of gaining business advantage.

Advice to employers

Employers who apply their own fitness criteria for work-related driving may seek information

---

Working hours

1. Drivers of large vehicles
European Union (Regulation 3820/85) and UK rules (Transport Act 1968, as amended) restrict the hours that a driver of large vehicles can spend behind the wheel. Most goods vehicles over 3.5 tonnes and around half of all buses and coaches are covered by the European Union rules, which require a tachograph to be fitted. Those exempted, mainly because of their type of operation and the distance travelled, are covered by UK rules which rely on records in log books.

Both sets specify, with some variations by type of vehicle and pattern of duties:

- maximum period of continuous driving (EU 4½ hours, UK 5½ hours)
- length of break (EU 45 minutes, UK 30 minutes) required before resuming
- daily driving limits (EU 9 hours, UK 10 hours)
- rest periods between daily driving duties (EU 11 hours, UK 10 hours)

- weekly or fortnightly rest breaks (EU 45 hours, UK 24 hours).

2. Others who drive for work
The hours of workers who drive smaller vehicles, as well as other employed travelling staff, are regulated (Road Transport [Working Time] Regulations 2005: SI 2005/639). These implement the European Union working time rules for mobile workers (Directive 2002/15/EC). The self-employed are excluded from these rules until 2009.

- average working week not to exceed 48 hours averaged over a 17-week reference period
- <60 hours in any working week
- not >10 hours in a 24-hour period if night work is performed
- there are also requirements for the maximum time without a rest break and daily and weekly rest requirements.

or advice from health professionals about individuals. They may also have access to their own sources of health advice, either in-house, through contracted occupational health providers or from published material. Health professionals need to take care when providing information or advice about an individual. The normal rules of informed consent apply. Key to this is a clear understanding of how any information provided may be used and what the implications for the employee may be. Where there is another health professional acting as company adviser, you may be able to discuss this with them. In other circumstances it is good practice to seek information from the employer on the policy and standards to be applied and to give information in terms of whether the individual meets these standards, if these appear reasonable, rather than in terms of a clinical diagnosis.

If you are asked to act on behalf of an employer, either to develop a policy on work-related driving or to advise on compliance with the clinical criteria of an existing one, remember that the topic is one that potentially brings the livelihoods of employees into conflict with a corporate policy. Hence ensure that you are competent to give such advice and recognize that your credentials are likely to be questioned in the event of a legally disputed decision.

Guidance on work-related driving

There is joint Department for Transport/HSE guidance on this topic.[7] Also a network exists of people concerned with improving standards of work-related driving, who can provide help – the Occupational Road Safety Alliance (www.orsa.org.uk). A number of large organizations have detailed policies on driving at work which apply to employees driving cars, vans, trucks or buses. These can serve as useful models for others developing their own policies and risk management procedures.

Summary

- The requirements of fitness to drive on public roads can be supplemented by management of driving risks by employers.

- For driving limited to worksites, employers often follow or adapt the DVLA standards for fitness to drive on public roads.

- There is great diversity in the risks and performance requirements for driving tasks at work.

- Requirements for equity in employment, as well as valid judgements about fitness to drive, have to be observed.

- Driving for work is subject to the same stresses and pressures as other facets of working life and these can affect driving behaviour and road safety.

References

1. *An In-Depth Study of Work-Related Road Traffic Accidents*. Road Safety Report No 58. London: Department for Transport, 2005. www.dft.gov.uk/stellent/groups/dft_rdsafety/documents/page/dft_rdsafety_039943.pdf

2. www.devonline.gov.uk/index/information_and_services/environmental_health/eh-healthandsafety-intro/eh-hs-guidance/eh-hs-forklifttrucks.htm

3. Lynn P, Lockwood CR. *The Accident Liability of Company Car Drivers*. Transport Research Laboratory Report 317. Transport Research Laboratory, 1998.

4. Jones GC, Frier BM. Medical assessment for licensing of taxi drivers by Scottish local authorities. *Occup Med* 1997; **47**: 40–44.

5. Booklet HS(G)6: *Safety in Working with Lift Trucks*. Approved Code of Practice and Supplementary Guidance, Rider Operated Lift Trucks – Operator Training. HSE. www.hse.gov.uk/workplacetransport/information/organising.htm

6. *Jones v Post Office* 2001 EWCA Civ 558.

7. *Driving at Work: Managing Work-Related Road Safety*. INDG 382. Department for Transport/Health and Safety Executive, 2003.

SECTION 2: SENSORY IMPAIRMENT

Vision is the dominant sensory input to the task of driving. The eye has to function under a wide range of lighting conditions, which may vary rapidly. As the visual information needed to drive safely is often transient and is moving in relation to the driver, this requires the eye not just to receive a stable image but to work in an integrated way with the brain, directing gaze where there are hints of danger and providing the information needed so that the road can be followed, and the speeds, directions and even intentions of other road users can be computed reliably.

Vehicle design and road layout can play an important part in determining the visual demands of driving. Headlights and a clean windscreen aid forward vision. Pillars and loads can reduce all-round vision, while well-placed mirrors can mitigate these reductions. Near vision is needed for instruments, with clear design minimizing the difficulties of adaptation and distraction from the road. Good road lighting, clear signs and simple junctions can all reduce errors from any vision or visual–perceptual limitations.

Auditory information can warn of dangers from other vehicles and of emergency services. It can also provide, usually subconscious, cues on the state of the vehicle and the road.

Inertial inputs received through the semicircular canals, through pressure against seats and through controls, assist with adjusting the pace and direction of travel.

Proprioceptive information and touch aid good use of the controls by providing feedback on steering. They also help with locating and using the foot pedals.

8. Vision

Impairment and risk
Clinical assessment and advice

Impairment and risk

Visual function plays an essential role as the major source of information about the surroundings of the vehicle. Several facets of eye function are relevant:

● visual acuity (distance and near) with or without correction

● field of vision, including discrete areas of loss of vision (scotomas)

● low-light vision and dark adaptation

● contrast sensitivity

● susceptibility to glare.

When an individual is driving, as in most other visual tasks, they use foveal (central) vision as a directed gaze for discrimination of detail. Their outer peripheral vision acts mainly to alert them to their surroundings and to direct gaze, while the areas between are used for a mix of functions. Most of the time the driver's gaze is directed to the road ahead, with periodic glances to instruments or to mirrors. The driver also identifies potential problems either at a distance, when they are in central vision, or because of peripheral alerting signals. These include movements, brightness or the shape or pattern of an object that is expected to pose a risk. The brain has to prioritize the use of gaze, and many of the skills of reading the road, whether taught or based on experience, relate to the best use of different parts of the visual field and the correct interpretation and anticipation of events.

The eye is only the first stage of the pathway for the interpretation of visual information. Innate and learned cognitive processes play a major part, and errors in them are also significant contributors to road accident risk. For example, the ability to perceive and realize the significance of a cyclist when the driver is looking for a car, or to divide attention among different sources of visual information and prioritize their importance when approaching a roundabout, can be an important determinant of safe driving (see Chapter 10).

Many of the more common causes of visual impairment are associated with ageing, and most of them lead to stable or slowly progressive functional limitations. More than one visually-impairing condition is not uncommonly found in the same person. The speed and quality of information processing also reduce with age. As a consequence the overall ability of older drivers to see and respond to visual information may be reduced in ways that are complex and hard to predict.

There are some links between diagnostic categories of eye disease and the form of impairment. However, in conditions such as glaucoma, macular degeneration and cataract several aspects of vision can be affected. Refractive defects, the most common impairment, are associated with loss of visual acuity, but with increasing age both corrected and uncorrected defects may be further impaired by the early stages of other conditions. While visual acuity and fields of vision can readily be tested, it is the subjective recognition of other problems by the driver, eg the effects of glare from increased light scatter within the ageing lens, loss of contrast sensitivity and reduced vision from poor dark adaptation during night driving, that is the norm (Plates 1–4).

Evidence – vision in general

● The quality of evidence linking different types of functional impairment with increasing risk is limited and rarely provides the sort of information that can be used to produce a clear dividing line between safe and unsafe levels of impairment. Much of it comprises comparisons between those who have and those who do not have a specific diagnosis.[1–4]

- Investigations of the risk to road safety from visual impairments are limited by their association with other aspects of ageing, by the frequent presence of multiple pathologies, by the selection out of the most severe cases during licensing and, most importantly, by the actions taken by those with subjective visual difficulties to avoid driving under conditions where these are found to interfere with driving.
- Studies have looked at crash experience, traffic violations and driving performance. For cataract there is some evidence of an increased crash and violation risk, but the evidence on other conditions on the road is equivocal.[1,5]
- Reduced visual acuity, as measured on Snellen and similar test charts, is only weakly correlated with crash risk and there is little evidence that measures of dynamic visual acuity are any better.
- Some measures of visual function, namely contrast sensitivity, and/or visual attention, such as the useful field of view test, which are not routinely used in visual assessments for driving, have shown associations with crash risk and poor driving performance.[5]
- Simulator studies do show some changes in performance associated with most of the main conditions and with visual function, but the road safety implications of the changes are unclear.

A number of conditions cause reductions in visual acuity, while for others the predominant feature is a reduction in the fields of vision. Some present with a mixed picture.

Refractive errors and reduced visual acuity

Visual acuity is most commonly reduced by errors in the refractive functions of the eyes. Reduced visual acuity is also a predominant feature of cataracts, macular degeneration and corneal disease. Diabetic eye disease may present with both refractive errors and defects of the fields of vision. Near vision is needed for reading maps and in-car instruments, but it is the quality of distant vision that is crucial to driving performance. Distance vision is normally tested in terms of central (foveal) performance, under good lighting conditions and using stationary symbols. The ability to detect movement and other visual clues anywhere in the visual fields, to respond to them by coordinating eye movements and to analyse their significance is essential for safe driving. Other normally untested but relevant aspects are acuity in low light conditions and the presence of glare.[6,7]

Evidence – refraction and visual acuity

- The relationship between visual acuity and road safety is not established in detail, as most visual defects are reduced by the assessment of refractive error and the use of corrective glasses or contact lenses. Those with more extreme defects have always been excluded from driving.[1]
- Corrective lenses for large refractive errors can narrow the field of view, as can thick frames. More recent devices for correcting major reductions in visual acuity function include small telescopes (bioptics). While these may increase visual acuity in the foveal region, they do this at the expense of the field of vision and also create a ring scotoma where there is no vision around the magnified area.[3]
- Refractive surgery to the cornea can provide improvements in visual acuity without the need for external visual correction. Increased glare sensitivity and a reduction in low-light contrast sensitivity

These plates provide an indication of the effects of different forms of visual loss on vision at the wheel. Visual loss is not easily simulated as the brain can, to an extent, use images from the better eye as well as eye and head movement to reduce the effects of loss of vision from parts of the visual field. Also, because of the way in which the brain analyses visual information, localized loss of visual function may not be subjectively apparent.

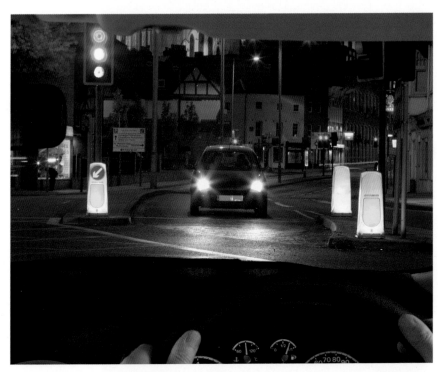

Plate 1: City driving on a clear night – light signals, signs, other road markings and road users readily apparent.

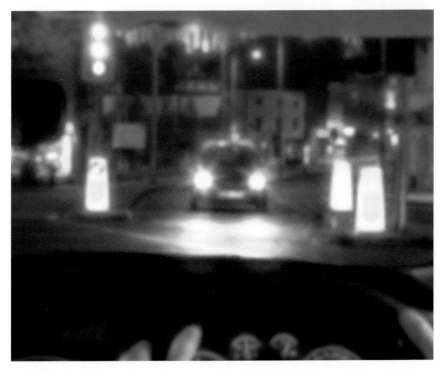

Plate 2: City driving on a clear night in a person with reduced visual acuity and increased light scatter in eye. Common in older drivers with early cataracts – loss of clarity because of glare, some signs no longer visible.

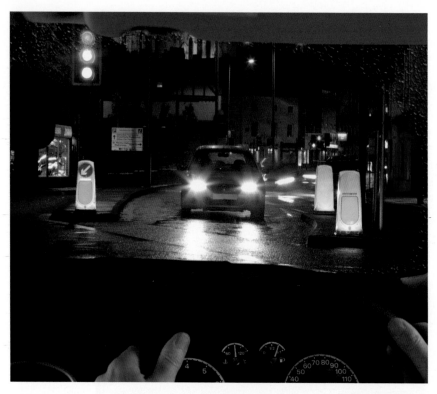

Plate 3: City driving on wet night – increased reflections and glare from water on road and windscreen. Some loss of information.

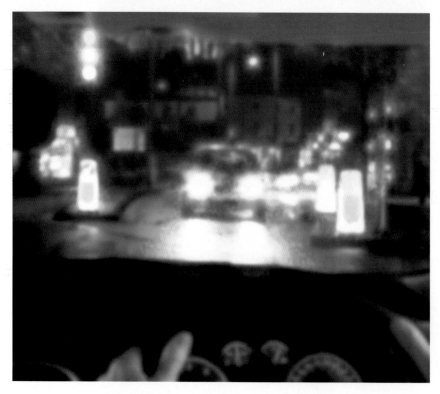

Plate 4: City driving on wet night in a person with reduced visual acuity and increased light scatter in eye. Common in older drivers with early cataracts – marked loss of clarity, road layout not visible, signs not apparent.

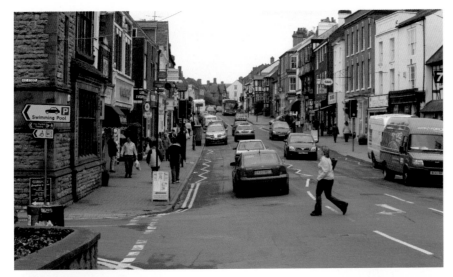

Plate 5: Street scene – normal vision

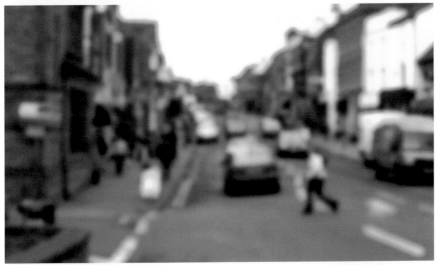

Plate 6: Cataract – loss of acuity and change to colour rendering

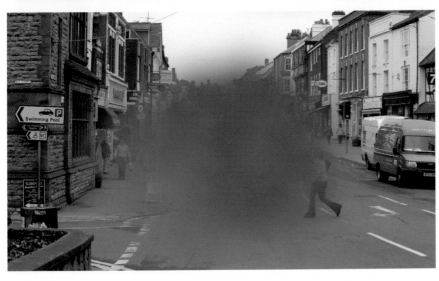

Plate 7: Macular degeneration – loss of central vision

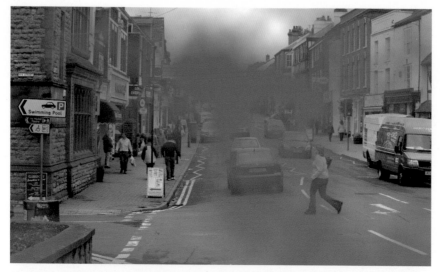

Plate 8: Diabetic retinopathy – patchy loss of vision across field

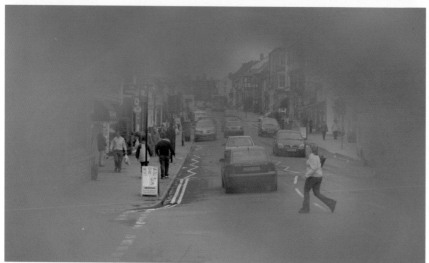

Plate 9: Glaucoma – mainly loss of peripheral vision

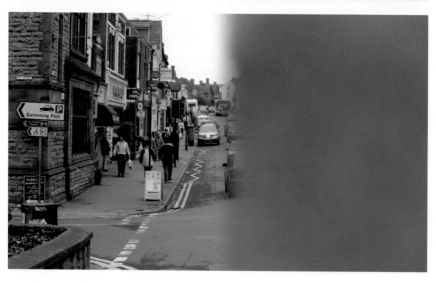

Plate 10: Hemianopia – loss of a large segment of visual field

are not uncommon after treatment. While the former usually resolves or can be managed with sunglasses, the latter can sometimes persist, although not normally to the extent that driving needs to be stopped or limited.[8]

- The frequency of refractive errors increases with age, as hardening of the human lens leads to limited accommodation and presbyopia. A number of studies show that unrecognized visual acuity defects, mainly loss of distance vision, are the most common abnormality found when screening drivers over 50 years of age for health-related impairments to driving. Defects in refraction are so common that they will often complicate the visual performance of people with other forms of eye disease.[2,4]

Cataract

The majority of cataracts that interfere with visual function are in older drivers. The progressive opacity of the human lens is usually bilateral. The diffuse scatter of light from the opaque lens reduces acuity and contrast sensitivity; it also increases the susceptibility of the eye to glare from bright light sources. All these have the potential to reduce driving performance, but glare at night or from the low sun causing temporary impairment to vision are particularly common problems in the early stages of cataract (Plates 1–6).

Evidence – cataract[1,9]

- Surgery provides a good restoration of function. In most cases it is not performed until there is a marked decline in vision; hence those with early-stage cataracts will have a period with some impairment to their visual function as drivers prior to surgery. Post surgery there is evidence of a reduction in crash risk.
- Five-year follow-up confirms the maintenance of improved visual function.[10]
- There has been more investigation of the effects of cataract on driving safety than for other eye conditions. An increased

frequency of crashes has been found in some but not all studies, and it has to be recognized that many drivers alter their pattern of driving to accommodate the effects of the condition.

- Studies of driving performance in those with cataracts and in volunteers with simulated cataracts created by wearing diffusing lenses show some reductions in competence, particularly in relation to peripheral perception. However, the conditions in such studies do not fully replicate driving on public roads.

Macular degeneration[1]

Reduction in central vision from any cause will lead to loss of information on fine detail. This will manifest as reduced visual acuity and as delay in response to visual information. Age-related macular degeneration selectively impairs central vision and may cause total loss of central vision. Population studies on crashes and citations are equivocal, probably because of other concomitant age-related impairments and because such loss of vision will be apparent to the sufferer and lead to modification or cessation of driving. Macular degeneration is progressive and often not amenable to treatment (Plate 7).

Corneal pathology[1]

Corneal damage, from any cause, can lead to a distorted or clouded image and increased sensitivity to glare. There is no information on crash risk after corneal damage.

Diabetic eye disease[1,11]

A complication of diabetes (see Chapter 20) can be a variable pattern of visual impairment. For driving, the usual problem is reduction in acuity either from diabetic retinopathy or from cataract. The pace of progression of retinopathy may depend on the underlying disease and the quality of its control.[12] There is evidence of excess crash risk but uncertainties about the ability of those with relatively stable impairments to adapt to them. Progression may be delayed by laser therapy to the retina, which if given early can enable driving to continue. Progression is variable, with or without laser therapy. Laser therapy can itself lead to a series of scotomas and to reduction in the field of vision; however, the newer techniques for laser treatment are far less damaging than those used a decade or more ago. Old treatments which used extensive pan-retinal photocoagulation often restricted the field of vision (Plate 8).

Glaucoma[1,13]

Reduction in the field of vision is the effect of glaucoma that is most likely to impair driving. The pattern is inconsistent but generally results in a reduction in mid-peripheral vision, sometimes associated with loss of areas in the central fields. Although drivers with glaucoma report subjective difficulties in driving, the results of studies investigating crashes and citations are equivocal. Studies of performance on simulators do show a correlation between loss of field and errors but no link to visual acuity or contrast sensitivity.[14] As with cataract, the condition is usually found in older drivers likely to have other visual or general impairments. There are particular difficulties in deciding the significance of measured visual field loss in an individual. As the condition is irreversible and damage is progressive, any impairment will almost certainly worsen over time (Plate 9).

Retinitis pigmentosa[1]

This genetic condition impairs vision, both by constricting the peripheral field of vision and by the loss of the low-light receptors or rods in the retina, leading to night blindness, susceptibility to glare and sometimes to major defects in peripheral and central vision.

Loss of field of vision – other causes

In addition to the causes noted above, loss of parts of the field of vision (Plate 10) can arise from conditions of the eyes, nerves and brain:

- congenital ocular anomalies, such as tilted discs, which can cause field defects and scotomas

- retinal detachment
- birth trauma to the brain or visual pathways
- stroke, the most common cause of hemianopia
- intracranial tumours, especially of the pituitary gland
- after cranial surgery

Evidence – visual field loss[1]

- The prognosis will depend on the underlying cause, as will the extent of recovery after sudden loss. This may be complicated by associated cognitive effects from causes such as stroke.

- There is evidence that adaptation and compensation for loss can occur where the condition is stable, especially when it occurs early in life. In the absence of cognitive impairment there may be scope for training to assist compensation.[15]

- The patterns of loss are very variable, with both the size of scotoma and its density influencing overall visual function, and with different effects depending on whether the loss is mainly in the periphery or the central field, which have very different functions. Consequently the effects on driving performance can be expected to be variable. In particular the part of the peripheral visual field affected is likely to have a major effect on which visual cues the driver picks up, eg are visual cues to the right, left or above the road noted and acted on. This also means that studies of crash risk or driving performance are of limited predictive value. However, in general, the more restricted the vertical and horizontal fields the greater the reduction in on-road driving performance.[16]

Monocular vision[1]

Binocular vision enables an individual to have three-dimensional awareness of their surroundings. This is important for near objects but provides little visual information about the position of distant objects, where the brain relies on other clues, such as parallax, to judge distance, motion and speed. Monocular vision and lack of stereoscopic vision are not uncommon and there is no indication of reduced driving performance in people with only one working eye.[17] However, as there is no second eye to compensate for any visual defect in the working eye, the working eye has to be fully functional and free from impairment. Also there are theoretical concerns about the limitations to field of vision, especially in situations like driving a forklift truck, where visual information has to be perceived from many directions as the truck is backed and turned in what are often congested locations. A driver will need a period for visual adaptation before driving performance is re-established following the sudden onset of monocularity. As well as the complete loss of function in one eye, it is not uncommon for functional monocularity to exist where the second eye has severely reduced visual acuity or a squint.

Colour vision[1]

There are no indications of excess risk in drivers with defective colour vision on public roads. In situations where there are unusual or complex colour signals, as on airfields, perception of colour may be relevant, although this has not been formally studied. Colour perception is not uniform, with only a few blue receptors in the foveal area but a greater predominance at the periphery; hence the limitations of blue as a signal colour but its value as an alerting mechanism for the presence of emergency vehicles.

Diplopia, nystagmus and blepharospasm

All these conditions may impair visual performance by creating difficulties with the stabilization, formation and hence perception of the retinal image. There have been no specific investigations of crash risk for these three conditions. In the case of diplopia the key consideration is whether the second image interferes with perception of space, distance and speed. If it is a new phenomenon, the driver may need a period of adaptation before their long-term visual performance can be assessed. Functional defects may be reduced by surgical correction or by patching of the less good eye – the latter method having the associated problems of monocularity. Nystagmus is frequently associated with reduced vision from other causes, and the overall capabilities of function will determine any risk. Severe blepharospasm can inhibit vision, and it may be erratic and associated with tension or fatigue. The level of impairment may be reduced by the use of botulinum toxin to paralyse the muscles in spasm.

Theoretical crash risks associated with all forms of visual deficit can be readily postulated but, as noted above for each condition, evidence about the level of impairment that significantly increases the risk of road crashes is missing. As there is very little indication from accident investigations to suggest that the optical, as opposed to the perceptual, performance of the visual system is a significant contributor, provided the driver is in compliance with the legal requirements, it is tempting to consider that these requirements are appropriate. However, this approach does not provide a way of identifying whether any of the current standards could be relaxed, thus enabling more people to remain mobile without increasing the risks. Rational decisions on vision standards are also made more complex by associated visual and non-visual co-morbidity, where the various risk factors cannot be summated to provide an overall assessment.

Clinical assessment and advice

- Assessment of visual function in terms of visual acuity and fields of vision is the main indicator of current legal suitability for driving.

- Any other defects in visual–spatial and cognitive processes also need to be considered, as they may determine a person's ability to compensate for any functional limitations in the eye.
- The underlying pathology will determine the likely prognosis.
- An individual's subjective perception of limitations in function can be very important, and there is considerable evidence that such perceptions, particularly of glare and other problems during night driving, may lead many drivers to alter their pattern of road use. However, people do not always recognize decrements in their distance vision which mean that they cannot clearly see distant detail.
- Defects in the fields of vision, except where there is rapid onset, are not usually perceived, as the brain has mechanisms for filling in the gaps in visual images using recent memory and extrapolation, rather than incoming visual information – a potentially dangerous pattern of perception.
- Many of the readily available tests of visual function had their origins as clinical diagnostic tools and are not designed for functional assessments. This applies both to normal visual acuity testing, which uses stationary symbols with high contrast and good illumination, and to visual field assessments, which do not sample the fields in ways relevant to the perceptual needs of driving or take account of personal adaptive skills used to overcome any defects.[3]

Because of features such as glare associated with cataract or the marked loss of acuity and central distortion associated with macular degeneration, these conditions often lead to reported symptoms. In contrast, glaucoma, with its mid-peripheral field defects, often does not. As diabetic retinopathy is a complication that requires regular surveillance, it is normally screened for as a routine part of disease management.

Acute visual defects from problems such as retinal detachment, acute glaucoma or corneal ulcer may present in primary care. Where these indicate a potential emergency or a need for referral to an ophthalmologist, the individual should be immediately advised not to drive. Less urgent, and in particular refractive, problems will be referred to an optometrist for investigation and treatment. If the standards for visual acuity (number plate test or Snellen equivalent) are not met, the individual should also be advised not to drive until vision is corrected to comply with the DVLA standards.

The DVLA lists criteria for:[18]

- visual acuity – based on number plate reading at 20.5 m for all drivers, supplemented by formal visual acuity testing and more stringent standards for Group 2
- cataract – in terms of visual acuity and glare
- monocular vision (Group 2 only)
- visual field defects
- diplopia (Group 2 only)
- night blindness
- blepharospasm.

The driver should be informed of their duty to report their condition to the DVLA if they do not meet the published standards or if assessment is required. When undertaking a Group 2 driver medical, the examining doctor is asked to provide information about these conditions.

As visual defects are common, can impair many aspects of living, increase in frequency with age and are often treatable, screening is justified. Visual defects should be sought in any individual who has another illness in which they are a known complication, eg visual field loss and visual inattention as complications of a stroke, retinopathy in people with diabetes.

People are frequently totally unaware of significant defects in their fields of vision. It is a matter of controversy how these defects should be handled when they are found by routine screening in people who have passed the driving test and driven safely for many years without being aware of them. The technique currently specified for field assessment in relation to licensing is the binocular Esterman test. This is an automated device, which provides a map of the binocular field of vision using a relatively high level of illumination. Some other techniques are accepted as valid alternatives.[19]

As such a high proportion of the population over 40 uses glasses or lenses, the majority of routine screening is undertaken by optometrists. The frequency of follow-up by either optometrist of ophthalmologist will depend on the prognosis of any underlying conditions. Licensing periods for those with conditions such as cataract and glaucoma will also be determined by this.

Advice to drivers on the implications of their vision for driving may be in response to reported symptoms, eg of disabling headlamp glare. It may follow clinical investigations that provide a measure of function or it may follow acute or subacute episodes of visual loss or disturbance. The main aspects are:

- *Driving behaviour* – avoiding night driving, concern about the effects of fatigue on vision, presence of a second individual to find the route. There is a continuing need to recognize areas of difficulty and to adapt to them, where this is safe.

- *Visual aids* – use of correct glasses, access to a spare pair in case of loss or damage during a journey. Reserve glasses in case of difficulties with contact lenses. Correct use of sunglasses and dangers of use in low or erratic light (eg tunnel) driving. Window tinting (there are legal limitations on this) and use of visors and mirrors are ways in which glare can be reduced.

- *Medications* – the effects of both eye drops and systemic medications on visual performance.

- Time to adapt to any visual changes and confirmation that visual standards are still

met are required after *eye surgery and acute episodes of visual disturbance*. These can arise from a range of causes, such as episodes of blepharospasm, corneal infection, allergies, iritis, acute glaucoma, demyelinating diseases such as multiple sclerosis, and eye or facial injuries. Retinal detachment and retinal vascular occlusion can cause sudden loss of vision in one eye.

- *Licensing requirements* – the need for the driver to inform the DVLA. It should be noted that failure to meet the number plate reading test is an immediate and absolute legal bar to driving until such time as this level of visual acuity is restored.

References

1. Charlton J, *et al*. *Influence of Chronic Illness on Crash Involvement of Motor Vehicle Drivers*. Report No. 213. Accident Research Centre, Monash University, 2004: 365–415. www.monash.edu.au/muarc/reports/muarc213.pdf

2. Charman WN. Vision and driving – a literature review and commentary. *Ophthalmic Physiol Opt* 1997; **17**: 371–391.

3. *New Standards for the Visual Function of Drivers*. Medical Working Group Report. EU Driver Licensing Committee, 2005. europa.eu.int/comm/transport/home/ drivinglicence/fitnesstodrive/index_en.htm

4. Van Rijn LJ, Volker-Dieben HJ. *Assessment of Vision Impairments in Relation to Driving Safety: A Literature Review*. CIECA, 1999.

5. *Safe Mobility for Older Drivers. IA2(b) Sensory (Vision) Deficits*. Washington DC: National Highway Transportation Safety Administration, 2000: 31–35. www.nhtsa.dot.gov/people/injury/olddrive/safe/safe-toc.htm

6. van den Berg TJTP, van Rijn LJ. *Relevance of Glare Sensitivity and Impairment of Visual Function Among European Drivers*. EU Project Report, 2002.

7. Slade SV, Dunne MCM, Miles JNV. The influence of high contrast acuity and normalised low contrast acuity upon self-reported situation avoidance and driving crashes. *Ophthalmic Physiol Opt* 2002; **22**: 1–9.

8. Chisholm CC. *The Effect of Laser Refractive Surgery on Visual Performance and its Implications for Commercial Aviation*. Paper 2001/4. Civial Aviation Authority.

9. *Safe Mobility for Older Drivers. IA1(b) Cataracts*. Washington DC: National Highway Transportation Safety Administration, 2000: 6–7. www.nhtsa.dot.gov/people/olddrive/safe/01a.htm

10. Monestam E, Lundqust B, Wachmeister L. Visual function and car driving: longitudinal results 5 years after cataract

surgery in a population. *Br J Ophthalmol* 2005; **89**: 459–463.

11. *Safe Mobility for Older Drivers. IA1(c) Diabetes.* Washington DC: National Highway Transportation Safety Administration, 2000: 9–10. www.nhtsa.dot.gov/people/injury/olddrive/safe/safe-toc.htm

12. Lui WJ, Lee LT, Yen MF, *et al*. Assessing progression and efficacy of treatment for diabetic retinopathy following the proliferative pathway to blindness. *Diabet Med* 2003; **20**: 727–733.

13. *Safe Mobility for Older Drivers. IA1(d) Glaucoma.* Washington DC: National Highway Transportation Safety Administration, 2000: 11–12. www.nhtsa.dot.gov/people/injury/olddrive/safe/safe-toc.htm

14. Szlyk JP, Mahler CL, Seiple W, *et al*. Driving performance of glaucoma patients correlates with peripheral field loss. *J Glaucoma* 2005; **14**: 145–150.

15. Coeckelbergh TR, Browwer WH, Cornolissen FW, Kooijman AC. Predicting practical fitness to drive in drivers with visual field defects caused by ocular pathology. *Hum Factors* 2004; **46**: 748–760.

16. Bowers A, Peli E, Elgin J, *et al*. On-road driving with moderate visual field loss. *Optom Vis Sci* 2005; **82**: 657–667.

17. Johnson CA, Keltner JL. Incidence of visual field loss in 20,000 eyes and its relationship to driving performance. *Arch Ophthalmol* 1983; **101**: 371–375.

18. Visual disorders. *At A Glance Guide*. Swansea: DVLA. www.dvla.gov.uk/at_a_glance/ch6_visual.htm

19. Vision. Appendix: Field of vision requirements for the holding of a group 1 licence entitlement. *At A Glance Guide*. Swansea: DVLA: Chapter 6. www.dvla.gov.uk/at_a_glance/ch6_visual.htm

9. Hearing and other sensory inputs

Hearing
Proprioception
Inertia and balance

Hearing

Hearing provides all-round information, unlike vision, which is restricted to the field of view. The driver perceives warnings from horns or from emergency vehicles and then directs their gaze towards the source. Drivers also, usually subconsciously, use vehicle information such as engine and road noise to judge speed and path-finding as well as to identify vehicle malfunctions. There are few studies on hearing and crash risk or other measures of driving performance, and their results are inconsistent.[1]

Deafness, even when profound, is not a bar to car driving because vision can provide most of the required sensory inputs. Visual input will be particularly important in the absence of auditory cues and its adequacy should be checked. The ability to communicate in an emergency, eg about the load carried and any hazards, is essential for Group 2 drivers, and so the DVLA needs to be informed about socially disabling hearing impairment in a Group 2 driver to check that the driver's speech is adequate or that an alternative device such as a MINICOM can be used in an emergency. Some national administrations do specify minimum hearing standards for commercial drivers.[2]

Proprioception

There are no specific standards relating to other modes of sensation. However, proprioception, touch and position senses are important for safe use of controls, especially pedals. They also provide important feedback on road conditions and through the steering wheel on loss of traction prior to a skid. If these modes of sensation are impaired, as in peripheral neuropathies or after a stroke, then you should ask questions about the patient's ability to steer and about accuracy of location and use of pedals. If only the left leg is affected, you may suggest the use of automatic transmission. Vehicle adaptation may also be possible (see p. 49).

Inertia and balance

Inertial cues are used to judge speed and safety on bends as well as during acceleration and braking. Visual cues can make up for most of the lost information if inertial changes are not perceived. However, some balance disturbances that cause misperceptions of movement, disabling giddiness and nausea can reduce performance. If these symptoms are severe, driving should cease (see p. 99).

One of the limitations of the use of a driving simulator to assess performance is the lack of realistic inertial cues. This can make adaptation to a simulator difficult for some people as well as sometimes causing severe nausea.

References

1. Dobbs BM. *Medical Conditions and Driving: A Review of the Literature 1960–2000*. DOT HS 809 690. Washington DC: National Highway Transportation Safety Administration, 2005: 19–20. www.nhtsa.dot.gov/people/injury/research/MedicalConditions_Driving.pdf

2. *Assessing Fitness to Drive for Commercial and Private Vehicle Drivers*. Australia: Austroads, 2003: 65. www.austroads.com.au/aftd/downloads/AFTD_2003_FA_WEBREV1.pdf

SECTION 3: IMPAIRMENT OF COGNITION AND NERVOUS SYSTEM CONTROL

- Processing and interpretation of sensory, mainly visual, information is essential for taking the decisions needed to control a vehicle safely.

- Action to control a vehicle is based on perceptions that have to be prioritized, as well as integrated with learnt knowledge of driving and with remembered details about the intent of the journey. This is a continuous process, with new sensory information leading to adjustments in control.

- Driver training, experience, patterns of behaviour (such as risk aversion, aggression and impulsiveness), interactions with passengers and other road users, as well as the effects of concurrent events on attitudes, all contribute to the actions taken.

- Muscular action is initiated to effect vehicle control, as well as to direct vision so as to maximize the capture of useful information.

These processes all depend on common patterns of nerve action and integration in the brain and the peripheral nerves. Many conditions can affect more than one aspect of the analysis of sensory input and its conversion into the actions taken to control the car.

10. Cognitive impairment and dementia

Impairment and risk
Clinical assessment and advice

Impairment and risk

There is much psychological information about driver behaviour and risk.[1] This covers perception and cognition of risk and decision-taking. Sex, age and a range of fixed personality traits, as well as factors that affect the state of the driver in the short term, have been investigated. Clear correlations have been found for a number of variables, but these have not been sufficiently precise to use as the basis for decisions on individual suitability to drive.

Evidence – impairment of cognitive function

- Changes in cognitive performance, with slowing of response times and difficulty in maintaining and switching attention, are associated with ageing, but follow very variable rates of decline (see p. 42).[2]
- Dementia and other organic brain syndromes can, by their effects on cognition and memory, result in poor judgement while driving.[3]
- There have been many attempts to study the relationship between dementias in older people and driving performance. However, there are major methodological problems in designing a valid study method because most dementing conditions are progressive and may occur in association with other pathology.[4]

- There is good evidence of deficits in driving skill in those with dementia, as well as evidence of an increased risk of crashes.[5–7] There is also evidence that in early stages of dementia the risk increases are no more than those found in young drivers or at the limits for alcohol levels, whereas when the condition becomes more severe the risk rises further.[8]
- Studies of progressive dementias and driving risk have not used uniform diagnostic criteria. There have been a number of attempts to evaluate the utility of different screening techniques alone or in batteries but, beyond the use of scoring systems using broad clinical criteria and of competence in the activities of daily living, these techniques have not improved prediction of risk. However, some evidence suggests that groups of people with poor performance in visual–spatial and executive functioning tests may also show impaired driving.[8]
- Rehabilitation forms an essential part of the process of recovery from a traumatic brain injury or major intracranial surgery. Driving competence, including the need for vehicle adaptations, may be one facet of this, and advice on the feasibility of driving and the need for any vehicle adaptations normally forms a part of the rehabilitation process. In addition, the risk of seizures will determine how soon after the event such drivers are considered fit to drive. Neuropsychological testing has identified a range of deficits in these groups that may be relevant to driving, but the two studies on crashes in those who have returned to driving did not indicate any excess. Both studies also included those with damage from strokes.[9]
- Relatively stable conditions, such as learning disability, autism, Asperger's syndrome, personality disorders and attention deficit hyperactivity disorder (ADHD), can influence the process of learning to drive and passing the driving

test, as can some of the impairments of dyslexia. Hence there is some initial selection into the population of drivers. There is little specific evidence on driving risks from any of these conditions, apart from ADHD. Here three studies, each with some limitations, all point to an increase in crash risk. An increase in police citation rates for traffic offences has also been found. In simulator studies there was no difference in performance, but there were lower scores on assessments of driving rules and decision-taking. Co-morbidity from conduct disorders and defiance may have influenced the findings.[10,11]

- Impaired cognition may arise from changes elsewhere in the body:
  —Acute anoxia and hypoglycaemia can cause severe defects, prior to incapacitation (see Chapter 16, p. 135 and p. 143).
  —There is impairment in the weeks following coronary bypass surgery
  —Cardiac failure causing tissue anoxia is associated with impairment.
  —Long-standing severe hypertension and chronic obstructive lung disease also reduce cognitive functioning.
  —The recurrent effects of anoxia in obstructive sleep apnoea may cause impairment of cognition, in addition to the well established risks from sleepiness (see p. 149).
  —Endstage renal failure, liver failure and portocaval bypass surgery all lead to toxic metabolites reaching the brain and reducing cognitive performance.
  —Hypothyroidism is associated with impaired cognition, which may not always fully recover on treatment.
- HIV/AIDS. There is no evidence of risk from being HIV positive in the absence of the AIDS syndrome, although cognitive impairment is a recognized complication of the latter. Early concerns about risks from AIDS dementia in safety-critical tasks have not subsequently been confirmed.[12,13]

Dementia – common driving problems
- Forgetting familiar routes and getting lost
- Confusion between pedals in stressful situations
- Situations requiring complex or fast cognitive processing may cause an individual with dementia to stop in traffic when there is no need to stop
- At intersections people with dementia may fail to yield right of way appropriately
- Verbal suggestions from passengers, eg directions, may not be interpreted quickly enough or appropriately for timely action to be taken

Cognitive processes may be patchily impaired and a number of complementary assessment methods are needed to attempt to assess risk in driving.[14]

- *Effective analysis of visual input* is essential. Direction and speed of movement and their consequences in terms of passing, turning and slowing all have to be computed and used not only as sources of information for control decisions but also for directing gaze to locations of hazard potential, so that these can be evaluated in more detail. Selective inattention to detail in some parts of the visual field can follow a stroke. Here tests such as clock drawing can identify partial visual neglect (see p. 146). Expectations from visual perception can determine what is seen and acted on while the unexpected is ignored – as in looking at, but failing to see a cyclist or motorcyclist when the driver's attention is focused on looking out for cars that are turning. The usable field of vision declines with age and this may be a contributor to slowed driving because search times increase.[15] Test methods that use dynamic visual discrimination as a measure, such as the useful field of view (UFOV) test, do show some correlation with crash risks and with driving performance. These tests integrate many facets of visual perception.[16–18]

- *Short-term memory recall* is needed to assess the immediate situation where traffic flows are complex, and the delay or uncertainty shown by older drivers at complex junctions may reflect this.

- *Longer-term memory* will hold information on route finding, on road-reading skills and on car control. The car control aspects of driving are 'over learned' and, as they have been repeatedly reinforced throughout life, they may be well preserved in a dementing mind, while other more recent memories such as how to follow an unfamiliar route are lost.

- The *optimum use of attention* is needed for safe driving. Attention has to be maintained and constantly re-prioritized to the current circumstances. At times it has to be divided among several tasks and should not be distracted by irrelevant information. Division of attention is a common problem with cognitive impairment. The driver's capability may be assessed by adding additional tasks to a test drive, eg counting roadside items such as lamp posts or doing simple mental arithmetic. Failure to stop the trivial added task and focus on driving when the situation becomes complex is indicative of a failure to prioritize safely.

- *Social skills*, such as making allowances for the behaviour of other road users, following traffic patterns, and remaining tranquil and reliable in adverse situations, also need to form part of the process of cognition that determines driving behaviour.

- What is termed the *'central executive function'* is the decision-taking process whereby all the different cognitive processes are integrated and form the basis for action. A continuing, and largely subconscious, process of prioritization of action based on the information received about the car, the road and other users takes place. This too can be selectively damaged, while lack of inhibitions, eg to impulsive action, can result in a dangerous driving style. Complex tests, such as the trail-making test (see p. 156), can be used to assess executive functions.

Clinical assessment and advice

Reduced cognitive performance is only to a limited extent a health problem in the narrow sense of being related to illness; there is a large measure of variation in cognitive performance in the 'healthy' population.

Clues such as self-care (dress, hair, timekeeping), awareness of the sort tested by the Mini Mental State Examination (MMSE) (see p. 158), as well as the comments of relatives and friends can be indicators of the more obvious features of severe cognitive impairment.

Several organizations provide advice on impaired cognition, dementia and driving, eg the Alzheimer's Society (www.alzheimers.org.uk) and Picks Disease Support Group (www.pdsg.org.uk).

The health professional is only closely involved where there are severe defects, such as those associated with specific categories of diagnosis or incidentally as a part of clinical management of an older individual. Many reductions in cognitive function are transient, eg those associated with alcohol and fatigue, while the age-related changes are only sometimes associated with diagnosable predisposing causes.[8] Situations where the potential effects of cognitive impairment on driving should be considered during a clinical consultation include:

- after a stroke or transient ischaemic attack
- following a head injury
- as a consequence of psychoactive or sedating medication, including general anaesthetics
- where there is systemic illness such as impaired circulation to the brain or late-stage liver disease that may cause anoxia or other toxic effects on the brain

- in chronic alcohol dependency – if, unusually, driving is still permitted
- most difficult of all, the old or middle-aged individual who is showing signs suggestive of the early stages of a dementia. Here a structured assessment may be a helpful guide to risk (see p. 158)
- where there is a specific treatment aspect:
  —if supplemental oxygen is needed in respiratory failure to reduce anoxia for other daily activities, then the consequences for fitness to drive need to be assessed. In particular, the need to carry a supply of oxygen and making use a pre-condition of continuing to drive also need to be discussed
  —if clinical procedures are used where there may be impairment from medication, deep relaxation or unusual physical or mental demands.

Progressive dementias

The recognition and acknowledgement of the early stages of dementia have general benefits in terms of providing the individual and those around them with an opportunity to come to terms with a whole series of adaptations.[19] Advice on driving needs to form a part of this process. In early dementia, when sufficient skills are retained and progression is slow, car but not large vehicle driving may continue, subject to the decision of the licensing authority, which may require a driving assessment or issue a licence of short duration.[20,21] It may be difficult to assess driving ability in those with dementia.[22]

Those who have poor short-term memory, disorientation, lack of insight or judgement are almost certainly going to be unfit to drive and will have their licences permanently revoked. Given the increasing incidence of cognitive impairment and dementia with increasing age, there will often be other health problems present that may impair driving. There may be advantages in assessing the extent of any dementing changes as part of a wider

assessment of the older driver and their fitness to continue to drive (see Appendix 1).

As many dementias are progressive, a timely discussion of the potential for loss of licence at an early stage, either with the patient or with their partner or other relative, may be desirable.[23] This can enable them to plan any changes, such as moving to a more convenient location or disposal of a car, rather than have to act in a crisis at a later stage in the disease (see Appendix 1).

The dementia associated with Huntington's disease can have a relatively early onset and hence poses problems for drivers of working age. Advice may be needed because of symptoms of dementia. As the risk of developing the disease may be predicted genetically, and as it may sometimes first present with other neurological symptoms, it is at times necessary to give long-term advice on lifestyle and potential limitations, including the likelihood that driving will have to cease at some future date because of the development of dementia.

References

1. *Safe Mobility for Older Drivers. IA2 (e,f,g,h). Memory/Cognition Defects, Navigation Errors on Road Tests, Discriminating Maneuver Errors on Road Test, Decision Making and Response Selection on Driving Simulators.* Washington, DC: National Highway Transportation Safety Administration, 2000: 40–45. www.nhtsa.dot.gov/people/injury/olddrive/safe/safe-toc.htm

2. Dobbs BM. Medical Conditions and Driving: A Review of the Literature 1960–2000. DOT HS 809 690. Washington, DC: National Highway Transportation Safety Administration, 2005: 115–119. www.nhtsa.dot.gov/people/injury/research/MedicalConditions_Driving.pdf

3. Charlton J, *et al. Influence of Chronic Illness on Crash Involvement of Motor Vehicle Drivers.* Report No. 213. Accident Research Centre, Monash University, 2004: 109–120. www.monash.edu.au/muarc/reports/muarc213.pdf

4. Holland C, Handley S, Feetam C. *Older Drivers, Illness and Medication.* Research Report 39, London: Department for Transport, 2003. www.dft.gov.uk/stellent/groups/dft_rdsafety/documents/divisionhomepage/030261.hcsp

5. Dubinsky RM, Stein AC, Lyons K. Practice parameter: risk of driving and Alzheimer's disease (an evidence based review). *Neurology* 2000; **54**: 2205–2211.

6. Uc EY, *et al*. Driver route-following and safety errors in early Alzheimer disease. *J Neurol Neurosurg Psychiatry* 2005; **76**: 764-768.

7. *Safe Mobility for Older Drivers. IA1(a) Dementia*. Washington, DC: National Highway Transportation Safety Administration, 2000: 3–6. www.nhtsa.dot.gov/people/injury/olddrive/safe/safe-toc.htm

8. Brown LB, Ott BR. Driving and dementia: a review of the literature. *J Geriatr Psychiatry Neurol* 2004; **17**: 232–240.

9. Charlton J, *et al*. *Influence of Chronic Illness on Crash Involvement of Motor Vehicle Drivers*. Report No. 213. Accident Research Centre, Monash University, 2004: 127–132. www.monash.edu.au/muarc/reports/muarc213.pdf

10. ibid: 294–307.

11. Barkley RA. Driving impairments in teens and adults with attention deficit/hyperactivity disorder. *Psychiatr Clin North Am* 2004; **27**: 233–260.

12. www.alzheimers.org.uk/Facts_about_dementia/What_is_dementia/info_aids.htm

13. *Assessing Fitness to Drive for Commercial and Private Vehicle Drivers*. Australia: Austroads Inc, 2003: 66. www.austroads.com.au/aftd/downloads/AFTD_2003_FA_WEBREV1.pdf

14. Palmer K, Backman L, Winblad B, Fratiglioni L. Detection of Alzheimer's disease and dementia in the preclinical phase: population based cohort study. *BMJ* 2003; **326**: 245–247.

15. Roge J, Pebayle T, Campagne A, Muzat A. Useful visual field reduction as a function of age and risk of accident in simulated car driving. *Invest Ophthalmol Vis Sci* 2005; **46**: 1774–1779.

16. Owsley C. Vision and driving in the elderly. *Optom Vis Sci* 1994; **71**: 727–735.

17. Myers RS, Ball KK, Kalina TD, *et al*. Relation of useful field of view and other screening tests to on-road driving performance. *Percept Mot Skills* 2000; **91**: 279–290.

18. *Safe Mobility for Older Drivers. IA2(c). Defects in Visual Attention/Speed of Processing*. Washington, DC: National Highway Transportation Safety Administration, 2000. www.nhtsa.dot.gov/people/injury/olddrive/safe/safe-toc.htm

19. Woods RT, Moniz-Cook E, Iliffe S, *et al*. Dementia: issues in early recognition and intervention in primary care. *J R Soc Med* 2003; **96**: 320–324.

20. Impairment of cognitive function. *At A Glance Guide*, chapter 8. Swansea: DVLA.

21. Law-Min R, Cope D. Driving and dementia: roles and responsibilities. *Geriatr Med* 2004: **May**: 17–22.

22. Byszewski AM, Graham ID, Amos S, *et al*. A continuing medical education initiative for Canadian primary care physicians: the driving and dementia toolkit: a pre and post-evaluation of knowledge, confidence gained and satisfaction. *J Am Geriatr Soc* 2003; **51**: 1484–1489.

23. *At the Crossroads: A Guide to Alzheimer's Disease, Dementia and Driving*. www.thehartford.com/alzheimers/105013final.pdf

11. Mental ill-health

Risk and impairment
Clinical assessment and advice

Risk and impairment

Diagnosed mental ill-health, including those personality disorders that are severe enough to come within a clinical-care framework, may lead to patterns of behaviour such as impulsiveness, indecisiveness, excessive anger, loss of or excessive risk aversion and changed levels of arousal, all of which can increase the risks of driving. All are also frequent among drivers without defined health problems. Such behaviour traits are likely to be more extreme and can be associated with less self-awareness in individuals with a psychotic illness where their comprehension of cause and effect may be disturbed. People with the far more common features of conditions such as anxiety and depression will normally have greater insight. Although anxiety and depression may alter driving style, the risks associated with misperception of risk are less prominent than in psychotic illness and are within population norms.

Psychiatric illness in general is associated with several specific areas of impairment that may affect driving, including:[1]

- impaired information-processing ability; this includes components such as attention, concentration and memory
- reduced sustained attention, ie vigilance
- impaired visual–spatial functioning, including increased latency of motor responses

- poor impulse control, including an increased degree of risk taking
- poor judgement, including a reduced ability to predict and anticipate
- reduced problem-solving ability, especially in a complex and dynamic environment
- indecisiveness, eg in those with obsessive–compulsive disorders.

Many of the effects relevant to driving are associated with alterations to cognitive processes either as a result of the mental illness that is present or of the treatment given for it.

Immediate risk will be associated with the present state of the individual, but the prognosis of the condition is also important. This is especially so where, as in bipolar disorders, there may be a phase during which disregard of risk is a presenting feature, often without self-awareness. Where there are paranoid or compulsive features associated with cars and driving, these can also be strong determinants of the form in which any recurrence may occur and can indicate the likely focus for early symptoms.

Co-morbidity is common in mental disorders, in particular anxiety and insomnia in psychotic conditions. Alcohol and substance abuse are other frequent co-morbid findings. These may have implications for safe driving that are more important than the diagnostic label applied to the disorder.

The more serious mental illnesses, such as schizophrenia and severe depression, carry a heavy load of associated personal, occupational and social impairments. The ability to drive a car may play an important part in the rehabilitation process.

Medication used for mental health problems can reduce the risks associated with driving that arise from the underlying condition but it may, by its effects on arousal, sleepiness or motor functions, create risks on its own account. Return to normal activities as soon as possible is a key part of the therapy for many mental health problems. Resumption of driving is an important aspect of this and will also often be a prerequisite of a return to work. Thus there may be inherent conflicts between the management of the condition for the benefit of the patient and the need to minimize road risk.

A wide range of impairments that could affect safety at the wheel can be deduced from the wider patterns of behaviour in those with mental ill-health. These include defects of attention, speed of information processing, fatigue, suicidal thoughts, aggression, impulsiveness and intolerance. Some of the studies of crash risk and citations show a small increase in groups defined in various ways as having mental health problems. Almost all these findings are skewed because the lower average mileage driven by most of those with mental health problems is not taken into account. The level of standardization of diagnosis, severity and prevalence is also variable.[2] There are no simulator studies.[3]

Evidence – effects of treatment

The effects of medications used for psychiatric disorders have been investigated in greater detail than the conditions themselves. Treatment effects are more readily investigated, especially by means of simulator studies. They are discussed here because of their close relationship with any risks of the underlying condition.

- *Antipsychotics.* There are no studies on the association between their use and either crashes or citations. These are the least studied group of psychotropic medications in terms of driving-related impairment. When treatment is started, the effects of sedation, poor coordination and attention are observed, but over time there are varying degrees of adaptation to and tolerance of these effects. A particular problem is the extrapyramidal effects of the older antipsychotic medications, which can induce tremor, involuntary movements and stiffness. Nevertheless, compared with untreated patients, some aspects of psychomotor performance may be improved in treated patients.[4]

- *Antidepressants.* One large study showed a doubling of crash risk in those on tricyclic antidepressants, but the variables such as car use and alcohol were not corrected for. Simulator studies with volunteers have shown marked impairment of psychomotor functions with most tricyclic compounds but fewer or no changes with selective serotonin reuptake inhibitors (SSRIs).[5]

- *Anxiolytics.* The most commonly used medications are benzodiazepines. Different products have big differences in elimination half-life, and this will influence the duration of any impairment. Common forms of impairment are sedation, prolonged reaction times, lack of coordination, memory loss, vertigo, dizziness and double vision. Several studies have shown an increased risk of crashes in those on benzodiazepines.[6] In one study this effect was limited to those on long-acting preparations. Simulator studies have been performed on patients, and these show multiple forms of impaired driving performance. Because of the study design it is not possible to separate out effects of medication from those of the underlying illness.[7]

- *Insomnia* is a common symptom in a range of mental disorders, and hypnotic medications are often prescribed. Hypnotic medications may result in impairments the next day, particularly early on, especially with longer-acting preparations. Tolerance usually occurs after one to two weeks.

- *Stimulants.* Two studies indicate that the stimulant methylphenidate used to treat attention deficit hyperactivity disorder (ADHD) may improve the driving ability in this group.[8,9]

- *Herbal products,* such as valerian for insomnia, can have sedative effects.

- There is substantial evidence that medications used to treat mental health problems have the potential to impair driving performance, but this needs to be considered in relation to any adverse effects of the underlying illness. Non-compliance with medication use may of itself be an indicator of potential risk-taking behaviour or lack of insight about the illness.[10]

- There is evidence of at least additive effects from the concurrent use of psychotropic medications and alcohol. Some side effects such as drowsiness are readily perceived, while others, like slowing of reaction times or problems in dividing attention, may not be.

Clinical assessment and advice

Clinical decision-taking on mental processes and fitness to drive is more difficult than for almost any other group of conditions.

- Diagnostic criteria are far from clear, hence there are few fitness standards that can be linked clearly with particular illnesses or forms of impairment.
- The present state of the patient may reduce their ability to have a rational discussion about fitness to drive.
- Insight may be limited or lacking, hence the patient cannot always be relied on to self-police their present state of impairment and avoid driving when subjectively impaired.
- Disregard of risk or an excess of anxiety or of obsessive behaviour may be a feature of the condition.
- Medication may reduce the risks from the underlying condition but, especially when newly started, can cause disabling symptoms that are not apparent to the patient.
- Encouraging a return to full activities will often be a part of therapy. Driving is likely to be an important part of this process and one where the clinician's best course of action for their patient may come into conflict with the safety of other road users.

It may be useful to consider the advice given in terms of:

- whether the patient can be expected to have the insight to decide when it is appropriate to drive
- what the needs are for directed advice from the practitioner
- if there is a need for the licensing authority to be contacted.

The patient's level of insight and how this may be changed by different phases of their illness or impairment is important in deciding how to proceed. The health professional will need to consider compliance with any treatment, sensible self-policing, and any requirement to inform the licensing authority.

The pattern of driving will also need to be considered. Drivers of large vehicles have to comply with more stringent licensing standards and some forms of mental illness may lead to a long period away from such duties. Those who drive as part of their work are likely to have less freedom to cease driving if their condition or medication is causing problems.

The DVLA lists criteria for:[11]

- anxiety and depression – severe with significant memory or concentration problems, agitation, behavioural disturbances or suicidal thoughts
- acute psychotic disorders of any type
- hypomania/mania
- chronic schizophrenia and other chronic psychoses
- dementia or any organic brain syndromes
- learning disability
- developmental disorders such as autism, Asperger's syndrome, ADHD
- behaviour disorders, including personality disorders, post head injury syndrome and non-epileptic seizure disorder.

Advice on common conditions

- *Anxiety or depression* without significant problems of memory, concentration, agitation, behavioural disturbance or suicidal thoughts. The condition itself is unlikely to be a risk. Advice should be given on likely side effects of any medication, including whether the patient should limit driving until they are stabilized on treatment. Drivers of large vehicles should be advised about any requirements to notify the licensing authority if the condition or its treatment lasts for more than a few weeks. Some employers require disclosure of any use of impairing medication by those driving as part of their job. They will normally ask the employee for this information but could contact the health professional for confirmation.

- *More severe anxiety or depression* – presence of significant problems of memory, concentration, agitation, behavioural disturbance or suicidal thoughts.

  Anxiety – relevant functional impairments:
  —decreased working memory
  —more easily distracted
  —less attentional capacity
  —increased liability to 'panic attacks'.

  Depression – relevant functional impairments:
  —disturbed attention
  —impaired information processing and judgement
  —psychomotor retardation
  —psychomotor agitation
  —diminished concentration and memory ability
  —lengthened reaction time
  —sleep disturbance and fatigue
  —suicidal ideation: excess crash risk shown in one investigation.[12]

  Cognitive impairments, particularly if associated with poor sleep, may impair driving performance. The risk of suicide at the wheel needs special consideration. With any appreciable suicidal risk, driving should normally cease until the condition has been stabilized on treatment. The licensing

authority may need to be informed and a return to driving will depend on its enquiries. For drivers of large vehicles, a condition of a return to driving is likely to be a specified period of stability and freedom from any side effects due to medication. For all drivers, any associated misuse or dependency on drugs or alcohol will need to be taken into account in the advice given and in any licensing decisions.

- *Acute psychotic disorders – any type*. Disordered thought processes, paranoid thoughts or delusions and lack of perception of risk can be expected to increase risk. Uncertainty about progression or recurrence means that a period is needed before the prognosis can be assessed. Driving must cease and the licensing authority should be informed. It is likely to require a period of stability, compliance with treatment, no adverse effects from medication and a favourable specialist report. Where the condition is unstable or recurrent, or where there is poor compliance with treatment, return to driving may take longer. For drivers of large vehicles a period of years free from problems, with medication adjusted to minimize side effects, is likely to be required.

- *Hypomania/mania*. These conditions (bipolar disorder) pose particularly high risks because of the association of increased recklessness with lack of insight and often denial of the problem. Advice for a first episode should be as for other acute psychoses, with an additional requirement that the patient should gain insight before a return to driving is permitted. If a pattern of repeated episodes becomes apparent, a longer period of freedom from recurrence and compliance with treatment is needed. Misuse of alcohol is often a complicating factor.

- *Chronic schizophrenia and other chronic psychoses*. Continuing symptoms, even with limited insight, do not necessarily preclude car driving. This is provided that such symptoms are unlikely to cause significant concentration problems, memory impairment or distraction while driving. Any psychotic symptoms that relate to other road users are particularly serious. If there are any recurrences, then the same advice as given for acute psychoses applies.

Schizophrenia – relevant impairments (while in remission):

—reduced ability to selectively attend to important information while ignoring the unimportant

—reduced ability to sustain concentration or attention

—reduced ability to perform in complex as distinct from simple situations.

- *Learning disabilities* – severe learning difficulties (defined as below average intellectual functioning accompanied by significant limitations in at least two of the following: communication, self-care, social skills, self-direction, functional academic skills, work, leisure or health and safety) are not compatible with driving. In milder forms it may be possible for the individual to hold a licence subject to passing the driving test. Only minor degrees of such disabilities would be compatible with driving large vehicles.

- *Developmental disorders*, including Asperger's syndrome, autism, severe communication disorders and ADHD. New drivers who have severe forms of these conditions should be advised to include this information on their declaration when they first apply for a licence. Impulsivity or lack of awareness of the impact of their own behaviour on others needs to be considered and may be detected in the course of learning to drive.

- *Behaviour and personality disorders* of all sorts are major causes of vehicle accidents, though most are at a level where they do not become medicalized. Where a clinical

diagnosis has been made, including of personality disorders, post head injury syndrome and non-epileptic seizure disorder, formal assessment is needed. Interactions with alcohol are a common problem. A licence would be revoked if serious disturbances such as violence or aggression created potential danger at the wheel. Patients may not be willing to inform licensing authorities of their condition.

Personality disorders – relevant impairments:

—aggression

—egocentricity

—impulsiveness

—resentment of authority

—intolerance of frustration

—irresponsibility.

Behaviour and personality disorders may contribute to a wide range of asocial or criminal acts on the roads, including:

—alcohol and drug-related driving offences

—'road rage' – acts of personal aggressiveness towards other road users

—car crime

—suicide and homicide on the roads

—dangerous and careless driving offences.

—driving while unlicensed or uninsured.

There are strong statistical correlations between, for example, a criminal record and failure to hold insurance.

References

1. Charlton J, *et al. Influence of Chronic Illness on Crash Involvement of Motor Vehicle Drivers*. Report No. 213. Accident Research Centre, Monash University, 2004: 271 (citing Metzner, *et al.*) www.monash.edu.au/muarc/reports/muarc213.pdf

2. ibid: 285 (citing Dobbs).

3. ibid: 277–279.

4. ibid: 279–281.

5. ibid: 281–282.

6. Barbone F, McMahon AD, Davey PG, *et al.* Association of road-traffic accidents with benzodiazepine use. *Lancet* 1998; **352**: 1331–1336.

7. Charlton J, *et al*. *Influence of Chronic Illness on Crash Involvement of Motor Vehicle Drivers*. Report No. 213. Accident Research Centre, Monash University, 2004: 282–285. www.monash.edu.au/muarc/reports/muarc213.pdf

8. ibid: 300.

9. Barkley RA, *et al*. Effects of two doses of methylphenidate on simulated driving performance in adults with attention deficit hyperactivity disorder. *J Safety Res* 2005; **36**: 121–131.

10. Edwards JG. Depression, antidepressants, and accidents (editorial). *BMJ* 1995; **311**: 887–888.

11. *At A Glance Guide*. Swansea: DVLA. www.dvla.gov.uk/at_a_glance/ch4_psychiatric.htm

12. Lam LT, Norton R, Connor J, Ameratunga S. Suicidal ideation, antidepressive medication and car crash injury. *Accid Anal Prev* 2005; **37**: 335–339.

12. Nervous system diseases

Stroke and transient ischaemic attack
Parkinson's disease
Multiple sclerosis
Other progressive neurological diseases
Peripheral neuropathies
Congenital and childhood neurological conditions
Liability to sudden attacks of unprovoked or unprecipitated disabling giddiness
Migraine and severe headaches
Acute encephalitic illnesses and meningitis
Transient global amnesia
Spinal cord trauma – paraplegia and quadriplegia
Intracranial trauma (serious head injury), intracranial lesions (vascular, abscess, tumour), intracranial surgery

(Epilepsy and seizure risk are covered in Chapter 17.)

Coordinated function of the nervous system is central to the driving task. In consequence neurological disease has the potential to cause a wide range of impairments:

- reduced ability to gain sensory information from the special senses and the body

- limitations in some or all cognitive processes, from the subtle to unconsciousness. Distraction from task by pain or other symptoms

- problems with car control because of weakness, altered muscle tone or uncontrolled movements.

These impairments may be constant, of sudden onset or fluctuating in severity, or may progress to increased disability or to recovery.

The present state of an individual's nervous system function can be assessed irrespective of diagnosis, by using performance tests and driving assessment, either on-road or simulated. Diagnosis will, however, inform present state assessment by pointing to the most likely areas of impairment. Prognosis is almost entirely dependent on the natural history of each illness. Most of the evidence on risk relates to particular illnesses, and so impairment, risk and advice are considered separately for the more common conditions. These should be used as exemplars for those illnesses not discussed.[1] For those conditions listed by the DVLA, summarized information on the main aspects of assessment and advice, including notification requirements, is given in Table 12.1 at the end of this chapter.[2]

Stroke and transient ischaemic attack

Impairment and risk

The pattern of impairment from stroke and transient ischaemic attack (TIA) is among the most complicated in terms of its effects on capability to drive safely. While some changes are apparent, others can be too subtle for the individual or their clinician to note without specifically considering driving performance:

- memory
- cognition – decision-making and executive functions
- attention – in particular hemi-neglect, with failure to attend to one side of space. The ability to divide and prioritize attention may be reduced

- visual–spatial perception, especially of moving objects
- speech and language comprehension
- vision – in particular hemianopia (see p. 72)
- sensory function – loss of touch and proprioception
- motor function – changed muscle control, strength, tension and balance.

Recovery of these functions after a stroke may be non-uniform, with subtle impairments remaining when the more obvious muscular functions have been restored.

TIAs show the same effects but over a short (<24 hour) timescale. Effects may cumulate if there are repeated events. The risk of both further strokes/TIAs and seizures is increased after an initial cerebrovascular event.

Because the pathological mechanisms underlying strokes and TIAs are usually the same as for other forms of ischaemic vascular disease, there is a raised incidence of cardiac events in those who have had strokes and *vice versa*.[3]

Evidence – stroke and transient ischaemic attack

- Studies looking at the relative frequency of accidents and citations have not shown marked differences between those who have had strokes and matched controls. However, post-stroke drivers will be a selected group. Only 30–40% of survivors resume driving, and driving habits may be changed by the effects of the condition.[4]
- There are only limited data on the importance of stroke as a cause of sudden death at the wheel. It is only likely to be subarachnoid and large intracerebral haemorrhages that cause sudden death; the time course for onset of incapacity from an ischaemic stroke is usually too prolonged. One study estimated that approximately 5% of sudden deaths were related to cerebrovascular disease, and cardiovascular

effects of atheroma predominate as the cause of sudden death at the wheel.[5]

- Cognitive test batteries are reasonably reliable predictors of post-stroke driving performance on simulators. Reaction times were commonly slowed.[6]
- Given the frequency of stroke as a cause of driving limitations, there is surprisingly little investigative work on it. This may well reflect the huge diversity of impairment that can arise, as well as variations in the extent and rate of recovery. Both will adversely influence the scope for valid methods of study design.
- There are data on recurrence rates and on the frequency of related conditions in those who have had strokes. A number of the studies based on large and representative populations are relatively old and their reported outcomes need to be adjusted to reflect modern approaches to treatment. More recent studies are mainly trials of therapy where a selected population is used, and so results cannot be extrapolated to the generality of drivers.[7]
- For TIAs it is possible to predict likely group recurrence levels based on analysis of risk factors, but the data are not sufficiently precise to use them to categorize individuals, except into broadly defined groups based on stratification of risk.[8]

Clinical assessment and advice

The main focus of such advice will be on the present state and its effects on safe driving. The risk of sudden incapacitation is only a long-term issue for drivers of large vehicles and, even here, it will probably arise from the effects of ischaemic vascular disease on the heart as much as on the brain; hence, a satisfactory exercise ECG is a requirement for a return to the wheel. Strokes with causes such as a one-off carotid artery dissection are an exception to this pattern of prognosis.

For car drivers, while the DVLA does not need to be notified immediately, a period of not driving is required after stroke or TIA. Then notification is only needed if there is residual neurological impairment, other than minor limb weakness not requiring vehicle adaptation. If there are repeated TIAs, the driver needs a longer period of freedom from recurrence.

While the effects of stroke and TIA on strength and movement are likely to be apparent, the health professional may need to look for damage to vision and cognition. The key to assessment is confirmation of the integrity of the loop of perception, cognition and motor action (see p. 3). Standardized forms of assessment, both in the clinical setting (see Appendix 1) and using more detailed test methods, are available.[9]

In the case of a stroke with apparent residual defects a full assessment is desirable, because the need for vehicle modification can also be considered (see p. 49). In those with a history of TIA and no apparent current physical deficits, attention should focus on visual fields and visual attention, cognitive and, in particular, executive functions, and stamina. In older age groups there will often be other functional limitations, eg to vision and joint flexibility. The overall capabilities, rather than just impairment from the stroke or TIA, need to be considered.

Residual impairments are often complex; hence a driving assessment (see p. 47) may be needed to determine either capability to drive a normal car or the vehicle adaptations needed before driving can resume. The driver may sometimes require tuition either to re-learn past skills or adapt to the use of novel car controls.

Parkinson's disease

Impairment and risk

The functional motor effects of tremor, bradykinesia, rigidity and loss of postural reflexes all have the potential to impair car control. Central effects, especially executive

---

Sequence for post-stroke/TIA car driver assessment

1. At time of stroke or TIA:
   —advise the person, if they are potentially capable of driving, that they must not drive for the next month
   —note if a seizure has occurred – if it has, then it may be considered to be 'provoked' but it may delay return to driving (see p. 130).

2. After one month:
   —assess the person's recovery and functional abilities, including cognition and attention
   —if the individual has made a full recovery, they may return to car driving. Advise them that they should initially test their own performance with short drives on quiet roads and then progress from there within any limitations they may have identified
   —if the individual has only residual limb weakness, recommend they try driving with another driver present, and that if they encounter any problems they should be referred for assessment of the need for vehicle adaptations
   —if other impairments are detected at the functional assessment, if the trial drive indicates that adaptation may be needed, or if any other problems are encountered, inform the driver that they must notify the DVLA and that they should not return to driving until the DVLA advises them that they can.

3. If notification to the DVLA is indicated, then check that the driver has done so and is not driving.

4. Respond to any requests for further information from the DVLA.

5. At the next appointment, find out about the person's pattern of driving, if it has been resumed, and their subjective feelings about any residual performance limitations. Give any further advice that may be indicated, including any scope for self-referral for assessment or appropriate choice of the next vehicle, and on alternative transport options.

dysfunction, visual–spatial difficulties and memory defects, can impair cognition, but these tend to develop at later stages of the disease, when reduced motor function has already limited activities. However, depression is a common associated finding at all stages of the disease, as is the beginning of sleep fragmentation and consequential fatigue and sudden sleepiness.

Medication used in the treatment of Parkinson's disease (PD) may also have its own effects on arousal and on cognitive and motor performance, not all of which are beneficial for driving.

PD is progressive, and driving is likely to be possible in the early stages, but it will then have to cease as the individual becomes more severely impaired.

Evidence – Parkinson's disease[10]

- There is good evidence of performance decrement in experimental studies associated with all the symptoms noted above.
- Crash risk is increased in those with more severe PD as compared both with controls and with those who have early-stage PD.
- Crash risk in those with PD is associated with poor performance on the Mini Mental State Examination (MMSE). More specific tests of cognitive impairment do not show a correlation with driving performance in those who are still driving or wish to return to it.[11]
- Both on-road driving and simulated driving performance in studies on those with early PD are worse than that of age- and sex-matched controls. Driving in urban conditions and in traffic flows is most severely affected. More severe PD is associated with a worse performance in the simulator study.
- There have been suggestions that some PD medications (pramipexole and ropinirole) are associated with sudden 'sleep attacks'. This has not been confirmed, but such attacks may well be an inherent feature of the disease.[12]
- A significant proportion of drivers with PD

themselves take the decision to cease driving because of their self-perceived difficulties.

Clinical assessment and advice

Because of the frequency of early signs of PD in older people and the variable rate of progression, advice regarding decisions on driving should be based on clinical assessment of the individual. Where a clear diagnosis has been made based on reported or observed impairment of the individual's ability to drive or undertake other activities of daily living, notification to the DVLA should be recommended, and in most early-stage cases car driving will not be limited. The DVLA is likely to seek further information on current disability as well as on rate of progression, and a decision will then be taken on whether to allow driving and on the length of licence to be issued.[13]

Several classes of medication may be used for treatment of PD, each with its own potential for impairing side effects. These may also exacerbate some of the features of the disease itself while controlling others, eg provoking sudden sleep attacks. Common impairing side effects are: daytime sleepiness, light-headedness, dizziness, blurred vision and confusion (see pp. 104–105).

Use of the framework for assessment (see p. 153) is a sound basis for deciding on the advice to give and on notification to the DVLA. The driver's self-assessment of the driving tasks that they find difficult is important additional information. If problems are specific to the use of particular controls, then vehicle modification may enable driving to continue. It is always important to consider whether there is cognitive impairment as well as motor limitation.

You should always ask about problems with driving in those with PD and, where possible, a shared decision on cessation should be taken when needed. Prior to this you can usefully give advice on where they should live and lifestyle to help the individual adapt to the condition and to their likely future inability to drive.

Multiple sclerosis

Impairment and risk

The erratic pattern of central nervous system demyelinization which characterizes multiple sclerosis (MS) means that both the pattern and time course of impairments relevant to driving are variable. A pattern of good and bad days may be overlaid on longer-term disability. Common ones are:

- motor abnormalities, weakness, spasticity, spasms
- sensory disturbances, in particular of vision and transitory parasthesia
- balance problems and dizziness
- fatigue – this may not be related to the severity of other symptoms
- psychological changes, including depression and, more rarely, euphoria
- cognitive impairment – slowed information processing, learning and memory recall problems, visual–spatial deficits, executive dysfunction.

Evidence – multiple sclerosis[14]

- The diversity of symptoms means that population studies will have only limited relevance to individual risk.
- There is no difference in crash risk between controls and those with minimal physical signs of MS but without cognitive impairments. Those *with* minimal physical signs of MS but with cognitive impairments have significantly more crashes than either of these groups. There are, however, no differences in driving offence rates between the groups.
- A cohort study comparing road crash hospital attendances in a group with MS and in controls found a higher level in the MS group. The number of attendances was small and it was not possible to correct for either mileage driven or for what determined whether to attend hospital in the event of a crash.

- No simulator or on-road studies of driving performance have been reported, but there is good correlation between impaired cognitive performance and poor results in laboratory surrogate tests for driving tasks.
- There are no studies on treatments for MS and driving.

Clinical assessment and advice

The variability of presentation and progression of MS means that assessment has to be on an individual basis. Particular attention to vision and to cognitive performance is required. The assessment framework (see p. 153) is a useful basis for giving advice. Where a clear diagnosis has been made, notification to the DVLA should be advised. Provided that visual standards are met and there is no need for vehicle adaptations, car driving is unlikely to be limited in mild cases of MS. The length of licence may be shortened to enable periodic re-assessment. For drivers of large vehicles licensing will also depend on the pattern of the disease in the individual, but with less latitude where symptoms vary in the short term, as vocational driving can rarely be adapted to such changes.

Advice on self-policing of fitness to drive is essential in a condition that can vary in its effects from day to day and where the pattern longer term is of remission and exacerbation.

Aspects of particular importance for safety are vision, disabling giddiness, muscle weakness and spasms, and variations in fatiguability. Bladder symptoms and control can also determine journey patterns. Where there is marked day-by-day variation, driving should be seen as a cancellable option and not as an essential aspect of life.

Early advice on transport options and on

maximizing mobility by location of housing should be considered so that progression does not restrict the patient's activity any more than is necessary.[15]

Other progressive neurological diseases (including motor neurone disease, muscular dystrophies, Huntington's disease)

The patterns of impairment will vary, as will the pace and variability of disease progression. In Huntington's disease, dementia may be the predominant form of impairment (see p. 84). There are no specific studies on crash risks or driving performance for specific conditions, but there are some relating to neurological conditions in general. These show a degree of excess risk.

Assessment and advice need to be based on the current state of the driver and on prognostic data on the condition. If the clinical assessment shows deficits that could be relevant to driving, then notification to the DVLA should be advised. The DVLA is likely, unless the condition is already advanced, to issue a licence of limited duration to enable periodic review.[16] Early referral for a driving assessment and for advice on any required vehicle modifications may be indicated. This is particularly important in steadily progressive conditions like motor neurone disease, as it is usually easier to teach the use of an adapted vehicle, especially one that needs to accommodate a wheelchair-seated driver, before there are too many limitations on movement.

Peripheral neuropathies

These may take a wide variety of forms and have a range of causes. Generalized neuropathies such as Guillain-Barré syndrome will usually make driving impossible until there is nearly full recovery. Advice on return to driving should be based on an assessment of current state, with the driver self-assessing their use of controls, first in a stationary car and then by driving short distances on quiet roads while accompanied, before returning to their normal pattern. Longer-term neuropathic conditions can impair the driver's control of a vehicle. These are commonly the result of peripheral nerve damage or a complication of diabetes. Referral to a mobility centre for assessment and adaptation of the vehicle may sometimes be needed (see p. 47).

Congenital and childhood neurological conditions (including cerebral palsy and spina bifida)

The common feature of such conditions is their presence prior to learning to drive. Many people with them will be able to drive, often in a modified vehicle. Specialized assessment and driving instruction will often be required. The extent of the individual's disability will influence their chance of success in reaching the required standard of competence. Success may be influenced by any associated learning difficulties as much as by the physical limitations imposed by the condition.

There is only very limited evidence about risk, and much of it focuses on the patient's training needs. For spina bifida, associated cognitive impairments have been investigated but found to be poor predictors of success in learning to drive.[17]

The use of a car can be particularly important for those who cannot walk any distance or access public transport. Hence it is important to see an initial assessment at a mobility centre as a key part of their care pathway in moving to adult life. This assessment will identify if any vehicle modifications are needed, the requirements for driving instruction and the limitations to be placed on the person's driving licence in terms of the specification of the controls that their car must have. The organizations supporting the care of those with such conditions are a useful source of advice on this, as are specialized clinics that provide continuing clinical management.[18]

Liability to sudden attacks of unprovoked or unprecipitated disabling giddiness (including Ménière's disease)

There are no specific studies on risk in these conditions. The driver should be told to stop driving until their symptoms are satisfactorily controlled. They should also be advised to inform the DVLA if the problem is a persistent one. Drivers of large vehicles must inform the DVLA on diagnosis. They require a period free from attacks, unless there is a totally treatable and non-recurring cause, before the licence will be restored.

Migraine and severe headaches

There are no specific studies on risk. Migraine and headache are unlikely to have a sufficiently quick onset to result in sudden incapacitation. Drivers with severe headache from any cause will need to plan journeys in a way that enables them to stop if necessary. They need to be aware of the sedating effects of some analgesics. Migraine may start with visual disturbance. There will usually be a short period when the vehicle can be stopped, but if migraine is severe or recurrent, then advice to restrict driving until effective treatment has been started may be needed.

Acute encephalitic illnesses and meningitis

The major risk relevant to driving after the acute illness is seizure. There is no separate evidence on these conditions and driving.

For drivers of both cars and large vehicles, unless there is residual disability or there have been seizures during the acute febrile illness or convalescence, a return to driving on recovery is recommended. The DVLA should be informed if any seizures have taken place. Driving should not be resumed prior to a DVLA decision.

Transient global amnesia

For car drivers a return to driving should be advised on full recovery, provided there has been no epilepsy, sequelae from head injury or other causes of altered awareness. If drivers of large vehicles experience more than one episode of transient global amnesia, they should be advised to cease to drive and to inform the DVLA.

Spinal cord trauma – paraplegia and quadriplegia

Returning to driving or learning to drive may be important for mobility. Assessment at a mobility centre and adaptation of a vehicle both in terms of wheelchair access and controls may be needed (see p. 47).

Intracranial trauma (serious head injury), intracranial lesions (vascular, abscess, tumour), intracranial surgery

All these situations carry a broadly similar pattern of risks and impairment:

- present-state loss of function: sensory, cognitive or motor
- variable liability to seizure or other sudden disabling event
- variable pattern of recovery or progression.

Evidence – intracranial trauma, lesions, surgery (impairing effects)

- After trauma, both neuropsychological testing and test drives are valid as predictors of subsequent driving safety, but the methodologies currently used are imperfect.[19]
- Tests validated for predicting the driving performance of people after strokes do not reliably predict driving performance after head injuries.[20]

Detailed guidance on common specific conditions is given by the DVLA.

If the individual has significant residual disability, such that they could find car control difficult or there is a degree of cognitive impairment, the DVLA will, if a resumption of

Table 12.1

Neurological conditions listed by DVLA: summary of assessment, advice and notification status.[2]

Condition	Clinician assessment specific to driving	Recommendations to driver	Notification to the DVLA
Chronic neurological disorders (multiple sclerosis [MS], Parkinson's disease [PD], motor neurone disease [MND])	Assess present state and prognosis Review known complications of disease, eg vision – MS, muscular control – all, cognition – PD and MS, sleep – PD. Consider assessment for vehicle modification*	Depends on present state: • if minor impairment only, no action • if fluctuating impairment, should not drive if subjectively impaired. At DVLA discretion if notified • if progressive, loss of licence should be prepared for. Refer if vehicle modification indicated*	Yes, once diagnosis has been established, on the basis of symptoms that are likely to impair activities of daily living and especially driving
Sudden disabling giddiness – Ménière's, etc	Assess severity and frequency of incapacitation and whether any warning	Group 1 – restart driving when symptoms controlled .... Group 2 – stop driving	Yes, if recurrent and not controlled by treatment .... Yes
Cerebrovascular disease (stroke, spontaneous intracerebral haemorrhage, transient ischaemic attack [TIA], amaurosis fugax)	After c. 1 month check for residual defects, especially visual field, cognition and serious limb impairment, or for recurrent TIA or seizure Consider assessment for vehicle modification*	Group 1 – stop driving for at least 1 month then assess: • residual effects • recurring events Stop driving until residual effects are fully assessed and mitigated Refer if vehicle modification indicated* .... Group 2 – stop driving	No, if no residual effects Yes, if residual effects, seizure, recurrences or if cranial surgery required .... Yes
Acute encephalitic illnesses and meningitis	Check if any seizures	No seizures – resume driving provided full recovery and no residual effects Seizures or residual effects relevant to driving – stop driving	No Yes
Transient global amnesia	Check if any seizures, sequelae to head injury or other causes of altered awareness present	Group 1 – continue driving in absence of listed risk markers .... Group 2 – stop if two or more episodes Single episode as Group 1	No, unless risk markers, then Yes .... Yes, if more than one episode
Tumours in cranial cavity – general (exceptions listed below)	Determine tumour type and treatment given Exceptions to general approach listed below Any seizure or liability to seizure voids exceptional criteria	Stop driving	Yes
Incidental benign untreated supratentorial tumour		Group 1 No action .... Group 2 Stop driving	No .... Yes

* See p. 47.

Condition	Clinician assessment specific to driving	Recommendations to driver	Notification to the DVLA
Pituitary tumour	Check for visual field loss	Group 1 – resume driving when clinically recovered (all treatments)	No, unless visual loss then Yes
		Group 2 • Craniotomy – stop driving for 6 months • Other treatment as Group 1	Yes No
Benign infratentorial tumour (treated or untreated)	Confirm absence of disabling symptoms	Resume driving when recovered, provided no disabling symptoms	No, unless disabling symptoms
Malignant intracranial tumour in child, no adult recurrence		Group 1 – no action	Should be disclosed on initial licence application
		Group 2 – individual assessment	Should be disclosed on first D4 medical examination form
Serious head injury (ie requiring hospital admission lasting >24 hours because of the head injury)	Group 1 – classify: • loss of consciousness, no haematoma, no depressed fractures, no seizures, no focal signs, no extended post-traumatic amnesia or residual cognitive or behavioural problems	Can return to driving when full and complete clinical recovery	No
	• serious injury no neurosurgery, no seizures	Stop driving (up to 6 months depending on recovery and seizure risk)	Yes
	• requiring surgical treatment for fracture, haematoma, etc	Stop driving (6–12 months depending on recovery and seizure risk)	Yes
	Group 2 – all of above	Stop driving	Yes
Intracranial haematoma (except when associated with stroke)	If chronic subdural (treated surgically)	Group 1 – resume driving on recovery Group 2 – stop driving	No Yes
	All other forms	Group 1 and 2 – stop driving	Yes
Subarachnoid haemorrhage	All causes and treatments with exception of normal angiography	Group 1 and 2 –Stop driving	Yes
		Group 1 – Resume driving on recovery	No
Truly incidental finding of intracranial aneurysm or arteriovenous malformation	Check no history suggestive of haemorrhage	Group 1 – no action	No
		Group 2 – stop driving	Yes
Intracerebral abcess or subdural empyema		Group 1 and 2 – stop driving	Yes
Hydrocephalus	Check if there are complications or associated neurological problems • intraventricular shunt insertion or revision	Group 1 and 2 – no action if uncomplicated Group 1 – stop driving for 6 months	Yes, at time of first licence Yes
		Group 2 – stop driving	Yes

driving is considered possible, often recommend an assessment at a mobility centre to determine capabilities and whether these could be enhanced by vehicle modifications. Where there are well established rehabilitation processes, as at major head injury treatment centres, driving potential will be one of the factors considered in assisting with a return to full and independent living. This will be particularly important if limb disabilities inhibit walking and the use of public transport.

Two of the more difficult areas for patients are where there is:

- *Reasonable physical recovery but cognitive impairment or disinhibition* leading to inappropriate impulsive acts, risk-taking or anger. Sometimes there is a lack of personal insight about these limitations and their implications for safety. As with other behavioural problems, health professionals may find that they need to go through due process (see p. 36) and then institute notification to the DVLA themselves in such situations.

- *A predicted risk of seizures*, and hence a restriction on driving, without one having taken place.

References

1. Yale SH, Hansotia P, Knapp D, Ehrfurth J. Neurological conditions: assessing medical fitness to drive. *Clin Med Res* 2003; **1**: 177–188.

2. Neurological conditions. In: *At A Glance Guide*. Swansea: DVLA. www.dvla.gov.uk/at_a_glance/ch1_neurological.htm

3. Witt BJ, Brown RD, Jacobsen SJ, *et al*. A community based study of stroke incidence after myocardial infarction. *Ann Intern Med* 2005; **143**: 785–792.

4. Charlton J, *et al*. *Influence of Chronic Illness on Crash Involvement of Motor Vehicle Drivers*. Report No. 213. Accident Research Centre, Monash University, 2004: 92–94. www.monash.edu.au/muarc/reports/muarc213.pdf

5. Dobbs BM. Medical conditions and driving: a review of the literature 1960–2000. DOT HS 809 690. Washington, DC: National Highway Transportation Safety Administration, 2005: 40. www.nhtsa.dot.gov/people/injury/research/MedicalConditions_Driving.pdf

6. ibid: 40–46.

7. Brophy S, *et al*. *Risk of Further Acute Vascular Events Following an Initial Myocardial Infarction or Stroke*. Road Safety Research Report 65. London: Department for Transport, 2006. www.dft.gov.uk/stellent/groups/dft_rdsafety/documents/divisionhomepage/030264.hcsp

8. Hankey GJ, Slattery JM, Warlow CP. Can long term outcome of individual patients with transient ischaemic attacks be predicted accurately? *J Neurol Neurosurg Psychiatry* 1993; **56**: 752–759.

9. Nouri FM, Tinson DJ, Lincoln NB. Cognitive ability and driving after stroke. *Int Disabil Studies* 1987; **9**: 110–115.

10. Charlton J, *et al*. *Influence of Chronic Illness on Crash Involvement of Motor Vehicle Drivers*. Report No. 213. Accident Research Centre, Monash University, 2004: 230–235. www.monash.edu.au/muarc/reports/muarc213.pdf

11. Radford K, Lincoln N, Lennox G. The effects of cognitive abilities on driving in people with Parkinson's Disease. *Disabil Rehabil* 2004; **26**: 65–70.

12. Homann CN, Wenzel K, Suppan K, *et al*. Sleep attacks in patients taking dopamine agonists. *BMJ* 2002; **324**: 1483–1487.

13. www.parkinsons.org.uk/Templates/internal.asp?NodeID=91811

14. Charlton J, *et al*. *Influence of Chronic Illness on Crash Involvement of Motor Vehicle Drivers*. Report No. 213. Accident Research Centre, Monash University, 2004: 244–247. www.monash.edu.au/muarc/reports/muarc213.pdf

15. www.mssociety.org.uk/what_is_ms/faqs/vehicles_or_mobility/driving_with_ms.html

16. Huntington's disease and driving. www.hda.org.uk/download/acrobat/hdafs013.pdf

17. Charlton J, *et al*. *Influence of Chronic Illness on Crash Involvement of Motor Vehicle Drivers*. Report No. 213. Accident Research Centre, Monash University, 2004: 252–260. www.monash.edu.au/muarc/reports/muarc213.pdf

18. Driving. www.asbah.org/Information/Driving.html

19. Keller M, Kesselring J, Hiltbrunner B. Fitness to drive with neurological disabilities. *Neurorehabil Neural Repair* 2003; **17**: 168–175.

20. Radford KA, Lincoln NB, Murray-Leslie C. Validation of the stroke drivers screening assessment for people with traumatic brain injury. *Brain Inj* 2004; **18**: 775–786.

13. Medication

Impairment and risk
Clinical assessment and advice

The effects of medications are also noted in some of the other sections, whereas in the treatment of mental health problems (see Chapter 11), seizures (see Chapter 17) and diabetes (see Chapter 20) medication and condition interact to determine the present state of driving capabilities of an individual.

Impairment and risk

Impairment from the use of medications, whether these are prescribed or purchased over the counter (OTC), is most frequent from products which have effects on the central nervous system and which interfere with cognition and arousal. A few agents impair visual performance, but interference with other aspects of driving performance is unusual. Common features of nervous system impairment by medications are:

- symptoms of drowsiness or detachment, sometimes with effects on coordination
- severity of perceived symptoms and measured impairment do not always correlate well
- there may be self-perceived adaptation to impairing effects. This may or may not be reflected in observed performance
- effects are usually but not always dose related
- time course of impairment depends on the product taken
- summation with other impairing agents such as alcohol and fatigue, which can increase perceived or observed effects

- interactions between the health problem treated and the medication, so that the balance of risks and benefits may be hard to establish
- interactions with other medications
- idiosyncratic side effects such as delayed metabolism, which may only be present in some of those taking the product, or where it may interact with a personal predisposition, eg to seizures.

Good studies on the effect of medication use on the incidence of road crashes and legal citations are rare. This reflects the methodological difficulties of designing them, especially in terms of correcting for the conditions for which the medication is given and the effects of both condition and treatment on the pattern of driving.

Evidence – medications and driving impairment

- Medications used to treat mental health problems have been shown to impair driving (see p. 88). Whether this manifests as an increase in risk compared with the untreated condition cannot be established because of the effect of most mental health problems on the overall pattern of activities, including work, social interactions and driving.
- *Benzodiazepines* have been shown to severely impair driving, when used as anxiolytics or as hypnotics. These effects are least marked for the latter when short half-life compounds are used at the start of the period of sleep.
- The effects of *insulin*-induced hypoglycaemia are well documented (see p. 143).
- *Narcotic analgesics* impair several aspects of cognitive function, such as attention and memory. They have been shown to impair driving when initially taken or after a dose increase.[1] Impairment may reduce with a prolonged stable dose.[2,3]

- *General anaesthetics* reduce cognitive performance for several hours after recovery of consciousness. These effects are not subjectively apparent.[4]
- A wide range of *OTC medicines* have the potential to induce unwanted sleepiness.[5]
- *Antihistamines*, used as anti-emetics, hay fever remedies and cough treatments, and to aid sleeping, impair driving performance. Some, especially the older ones such as diphenhydramine and chlorphenamide, are more potent than newer compounds designed to cross the blood–brain barrier to a lesser extent.
- The sedative effects of medications are potentiated by alcohol.[6]
- Sleep loss potentiates the sedative effects of medications.
- Subjective assessments of sleepiness and cognitive impairment from medication do not correlate well with measured changes.
- Tolerance may develop to impairing side effects of medications. This may sometimes be objectively demonstrable but it may also reflect a reduced perception of continuing impairment.
- Visual impairment is a short-term consequence of the diagnostic use of pupillary dilators. Impairment will also arise with long-term use and as a side effect when agents such as hyoscine (other than the non-absorbed hyoscine butyl bromide) and atropine are used for other therapeutic purposes. A few agents, eg the anticonvulsant vigabatrin, may have long-term side effects by reducing the field of vision.

Clinical assessment and advice

Labelling of medications provides information on risk.[7] Prescribers or dispensers may supplement this with further written and oral evidence. For prescription medications there are required statements to be included on the product label or packaging, as well as agreed wording in the enclosed product information leaflet (PIL). For some classes of medication there is required wording; thus all the older antihistamines have to carry a warning about drowsiness.

For OTC medications, while the PILs are standardized, the prominence given to impairing effects on packaging varies. Hence cough suppressant preparations of diphenhydramine warn, without prominence, that they may cause drowsiness. However, preparations with the same dose of diphenhydramine designed as hypnotics give prominence to their sleep-inducing powers.[8]

A few medications, such as the antiparkinsonian agents pramipexole and ropinirole, carry statements to the effect that driving should not be undertaken, at least in those who experience somnolence or sudden sleep onset. Most sedating preparations use the warning, 'May cause drowsiness. If affected do not drive or operate moving machinery'. This implies that self-awareness of symptoms is sufficient to prevent risk, a statement not borne out by laboratory studies of performance decrements.

All statements, the above included, apply only to the recommended doses. Should an individual overdose, say with an antihistamine hay fever remedy that is stated to be nonsedating, in order to control symptoms not prevented at the recommended dose, then sedating effects can be expected.

It is important to recognize and to advise patients who drive that medications bought outside the European Union or on the internet may not have similar warnings. In such cases the user should request information at the time of purchase or check with a source of valid advice such as a pharmacist whether precautions are needed.

The medications most commonly associated with effects that may impair driving are:

- *Anti-epileptics with sedating effects.* The dose may need to be maintained at sedating levels to ensure seizure control.

Licensing decisions on driving will primarily be determined by the seizure risk, but the prescribing physician will need to enquire and advise about sedation for some anticonvulsants.

- *Narcotic analgesics.* The severity of sedating effects is variable but almost inevitable. Timing of use to avoid driving with peak drug levels may minimize effects, but dose increases to control pain can have consequences for impairment. The use of maintenance methadone to treat opiate addiction is associated with impairment. In addition there may be risks from both increasing the methadone intake and from a return to use of other opiates (see p. 111).

- *Antidepressants.* Tricyclics such as amitriptyline and imipramine are more sedating that the newer selective serotonin reuptake inhibitors (SSRIs). The latter can cause some impairment, and caution is required when starting them or when dosage is changed.[9] The less commonly used monoamine oxide inhibitors, while less sedating than the tricyclics, have a range of other potentially impairing effects on the central nervous system.

- *Bupropion.* This was originally developed as an antidepressant but is now used at lower doses as an aid to smoking cessation. At higher doses it induced seizures and there remains a small risk at current dose levels. If it is prescribed to an individual with an increased risk of seizures from, for example, quiescent epilepsy or head injury, then they should be advised to cease driving for the duration of the treatment. Drivers should be advised to notify the DVLA if a seizure occurs.

- *Anti-emetics.* Can cause drowsiness and dizziness. Drivers should be warned.

- *Anticholinergics.* Many medications (including some antidepressants, antihistamines, anti-emetics, antipsychotics and antiparkinsonian preparations) have anticholinergic effects. These include blurred vision, sedation, confusion, ataxia, tremulousness and myoclonic jerking. Patients should be advised to cease driving and seek advice if they develop such symptoms. Subtle defects of memory and reasoning, as well as psychomotor and cognitive impairment of which the patient may not be aware, can develop. Users should be advised to seek advice if they note deterioration in their driving performance. Such symptoms need to be distinguished from the signs of early dementia in older patients.

- *Antihistamines.* Used for treatment of allergies such as hay fever, in cough suppressants and in some OTC aids to sleeping. Older preparations such as chlorphenamide and promethazine are sedating, while newer ones, eg loratadine and terfenadine, have only minimal sedating effects as they are less able to cross the blood–brain barrier. Users should be warned of the risk, especially when starting the medication and when dosage is increased. They should also be advised that severe symptoms of, eg hay fever, can in themselves be impairing if sneezing and watering eyes interfere with the driving task. For this reason finding the right preparation and dose of medication can be important if driving is to continue while the condition is severe.

- *Antihypertensives.* Few of the currently used preparations have severe effects of either sedation or orthostatic hypotension leading to syncope. If these are recognized side effects of the medication used, the patient should be warned of the need to be alert for such effects and not to drive if they occur.

- *Benzodiazepines as sedatives, hypnotics, anxiolytics.* Long-acting preparations frequently cause day-round sedation. Shorter-acting benzodiazepines have a half-life in the body such that a dose taken at bedtime is no longer causing a detectable sedating effect the following morning. Individual responses vary and there is a degree of habituation, probably both to the subjective feelings of drowsiness and to objectively measurable impairment. When treatment is started or the dose increased, patients should be warned about the increased risk of impairment while driving and advised to be cautious. Small doses of alcohol considerably increase the impairing effect, and users should be warned.

- *Stimulants.* For some conditions, such as narcolepsy and attention deficit hyperactivity disorder (ADHD), certain stimulants can improve driving performance. In experimental studies over-use or abuse to maintain wakefulness leads to increasing error rates and potentially to increased risk of a crash.

- *Insulin* (see Chapter 20).

- *Topical and systemic medications containing atropine or hyoscine.* Cause pupillary dilatation and paralysis of accommodation in the eye, increasing glare sensitivity and reducing visual acuity. Where these are used, short-term advice not to drive should be given. If they are used for a longer duration, vision should be checked both by questioning the patient about subjective difficulties and by testing acuity.[10] Absorbable forms of hyoscine also sedate.

Points to consider in advice

- *Clarify who is responsible for giving advice on medication*; do not assume that another party such as a doctor, pharmacist or specialist nurse will automatically be responsible. In a clinic setting where the same medication may be used frequently you should consider having a protocol identifying who is responsible for giving advice about driving, perhaps supplemented by an information leaflet for patients.

- *A higher level of precautions is required for drivers of large vehicles, in the emergency services and for some workplace drivers.* Employers, such as bus and truck companies, police and fire services, may

place additional obligations on drivers to report medication use to the organization's occupational health adviser or to their supervisor before commencing duty. If your patient drives as a part of their work, check if their employer has such obligations. If they do, then provide a note detailing the medication and its indications. If not, give advice yourself or offer to provide it for the employer and to collaborate if the treatment results in restrictions on employment (see Chapter 7).

- As there is considerable variation in response among individuals to many classes of medication, *the user has a major role in self-monitoring*. They need to be aware of foreseeable risks and how to detect them. They also need to be alert to any detrement in their own performance, such as lack of alertness, slowed thought processes or unsteadiness, as well as to an increase in lapses, errors or minor mishaps. If these arise and can be related in time to likely peak levels of medication, then driving should be avoided.

- *The dangers of overdosage should be emphasized, as should some of the rebound effects when medication is stopped*, eg lack of sleep when a prescribed hypnotic can no longer be justified.

- *Interactions between medications and between medication and other aspects of lifestyle*, such as alcohol use and lack of sleep, will sometimes need to form a part of advice on medication use and driving.

- *Drivers should be made aware that, in legal terms, they are committing an offence by driving while impaired from the use of prescribed or OTC medications*, just as they would be if they were impaired by alcohol. Hence it is their responsibility to refrain from driving if they recognize that they are impaired. Health professionals have been successfully prosecuted for failure to give such advice in other jurisdictions, and in Britain a dentist has been taken to court, but subsequently acquitted, when a patient crashed while driving after sedation for a dental procedure.

References

1. Bruera E, Macmillan K, Hanson J, MacDonald N. The cognitive effects of the administration of narcotic analgesics in patients with cancer pain. *Pain 1989;* **39**: 13–16.

2. Vainio A, Ollila J, Matikainen E, *et al.* Driving ability in cancer patients receiving long-term morphine analgesia. *Lancet* 1995; **346**: 667–670.

3. Chapman S. The effects of opioids on driving ability in patients with chronic pain. *Am Pain Soc Bull* 2001; **11**.

4. Edwards R, *et al.* Driving impairment following ambulatory surgery. *Can Anaesthesiol J* 2004; **51**: A71

5. Horne JA, Barrett PR. *Over-the-Counter Medicines and the Potential for Unwanted Sleepiness*. Road Safety Research Report No. 24. London: Department for Transport, 2001. www.dft.gov.uk/stellent/groups/dft_rdsafety/documents/divisionhomepage/030261.hcsp

6. Weatherman R, Crabb DW. Alcohol and medication interactions. *Alcohol Res Health* 1999; **23**: 40–55.

7. *Prescribing and Dispensing Guidelines for Medicinal Products Affecting Driving Performance*. ICADTS 2001. www.icadts.org/reports/ICADTSpresguiderpt.pdf

8. Horne JA, Barrett PR. *Over-the-Counter Medicines Liable to Cause Unwanted Sleepiness: Assessment of Package Warnings*. Road Safety Research Report No. 28. London: Department for Transport, 2003. www.dft.gov.uk/stellent/groups/dft_rdsafety/documents/divisionhomepage/030261.hcsp

9. Ward NE, Block E, Dye L. *Antidepressants and Road Safety – Literature Review and Commentary*. Road Safety Research Report No. 18. London: Department for Transport, 2002. www.dft.gov.uk/stellent/groups/dft_rdsafety/documents/divisionhomepage/030261.hcsp

10. *Installation of Diagnostic Eye Drops in General Optometric Practice*. London: College of Optometrists, 2005. www.college-optometrists.org/objects_store/eyedrops.pdf

14. Alcohol and non-therapeutic drugs

Impairment and risk
Clinical assessment and advice

Impairment and risk

Acute effects

It is the police who enforce the controls on the use of alcohol and non-therapeutic drugs for their psychoactive effects when they are likely to interfere with driving. Acute episodes of impairment are confirmed by measuring alcohol levels or by testing for either the presence of drugs or for their impairing effects.[1] Drivers at risk from alcohol and non-therapeutic drug use may also come to the attention of health professionals by way of the police or courts following a range of offences or behaviour patterns. They may be identified during clinical investigations for other conditions or following injury. Medical screening, either directed at alcohol and drugs or for other reasons, may identify markers of use. Unprompted self-reporting is rare.

Penalties imposed by the courts for road safety offences take the form of revocation of the driving licence for a period, the option of

---

Police procedures for driving under the influence of alcohol or drugs

(These are largely similar for road, rail, sea and air.)

1. Collision, moving traffic offence or suspicion of impairment from drink or drugs.

2. Stop the vehicle and do a breath test for alcohol:
   —if positive arrest, re-test at the police station and charge with driving with excess alcohol (equivalent to 80 mg% level in blood for road drivers, and for rail and sea workers; equivalent to 20 mg% for aircrew)
   —blood or urine tests may be used as alternatives where the roadside breath test results are borderline or where the individual is unable to give a breath sample and there is a good reason for this
   —refusal to give a sample is treated as the equivalent of a positive test
   —if the driver has failed to stop at the scene of an accident, the police may find them elsewhere and require a test.

3. Alcohol test negative:
   —possibly do 'Field Impairment Test' to assess performance decrements. The test comprises a series of simple assessments of cognitive performance and coordination and is being piloted by a number of police forces. (Not used for rail staff, except voluntarily.)

   —may be sufficient evidence of impairment without testing.
   —if test negative and insufficient evidence, then release.

4. If evidence of impairment from test or observation, then take to police station and call forensic medical examiner (FME), who will observe the individual to ascertain if the condition might be due to some drug:
   —if no, then release
   —if yes, then FME takes a blood or urine sample.

5. Send sample to laboratory:
   —if no drugs found in the sample, then no charges
   —if drugs found, then charged with driving while impaired through drink or drugs.

6. Once charged, the individual will be released and bailed to the court by the custody sergeant, but only when they are considered fit and not likely to commit a further offence (such as driving again when over the alcohol limit).

7. If a driver is at a hospital and is conscious, a doctor there may take a sample with consent, but bearing in mind that failure to give consent is taken to be the same as a positive test. If they are unconscious and so cannot consent, the sample must be taken by a doctor who is not clinically involved with the person. This will usually be a police surgeon.

attending a training course to reduce the period of disqualification (for alcohol) or additional charges for careless or dangerous driving. The illegality of use of controlled drugs also means that enforcement action is directed at offences concerned with use and with dealing.

If alcohol levels are very high, if there are repeated alcohol offences or if the driver refuses to give a specimen, then they become 'high-risk offenders' and come within the provisions of the high-risk offender scheme. The court should notify them that they are within the scheme. This scheme requires additional steps to be taken before re-licensing can be considered: a longer period of licence revocation, the option of attending a rehabilitation course to reduce this period, and a medical assessment aimed at detecting whether there is still a problem of continued high levels of alcohol use or adverse effects indicative of it.

For alcohol and for both therapeutic and non-therapeutic drugs the road traffic offence is driving while unfit through drink or drugs. If use is so long before driving that there is no impairment, as assessed by the levels present or performance, then there is no driving offence. Rates of metabolism and excretion vary widely, hence time periods cannot be specified reliably. Even in the absence of impaired driving there may still be problems from dependency and, in the case of drugs, other offences such as possession. However, the common patterns of use for any agent readily leading to dependence are such that regular users will not normally limit their driving to times when they are unaffected.

Health professionals may have patients with known or suspected alcohol or drug problems and need to advise them about driving and about the penalties for doing so under the influence of alcohol or drugs. They may also be concerned with those who have lost their licence for alcohol and drug offences and who wish to regain it. Specialist alcohol and addiction clinics may also be responsible for

the details of case management, including substitute agents such as methadone for opiates. They will also wish to reduce the barriers to employment created by lack of a valid driving licence.

Longer-term effects

The acute effects of alcohol are a common cause of road crashes, not only in those with alcohol dependence. The risk level correlates well with the measured blood and breath levels. These risks also need to be considered as a repeated phenomenon in those with the chronic effects of alcohol dependency. Dependency makes it harder to avoid drinking or drug taking and diminishes flexibility in patterns of use and abstention.

The longer-term cognitive effects from alcohol abuse include widespread and multifaceted impairment across many domains of cognitive function. Commonly these manifest as short-term memory and learning impairments, which become more evident as task difficulty increases. These effects are in addition to impaired perceptual–motor speed, and impairments in visual search and scanning strategies.

Evidence – alcohol[2]

- Long-term excessive drinking leads to deficits in cognition, especially executive functions such as planning and prioritizing tasks and attention, with impairment of visual–spatial judgements. Difficulty shifting and sustaining focus and inability to filter out distractions, as well as reduced self-regulation of impulsive actions, are common. Peripheral neuropathies may also impair sensory input and motor actions. Other long-term life-shortening sequelae, such as cirrhosis of the liver and oesophageal varices, are not directly relevant to fitness to drive, with the exception of encephalopathy in advanced liver failure.

- Elevated blood alcohol levels, even to moderate levels in volunteers, are associated with complex changes in cognitive and motor performance, which are not in step with each other – motor skills return more rapidly than cognitive ones as blood alcohol levels decline from their peak. It is not clear whether similar patterns occur in heavy drinkers who have developed a degree of tolerance to the effects of alcohol, at least on motor performance.

- The greater risk of repeated alcohol-related accidents amongst those categorized as high-risk offenders suggests that tolerance to the effect of alcohol does not protect against accidents. The self-belief among regular drinkers that they are better adapted to drinking and driving compared with the occasional user of alcohol is not supported by any evidence.

- It is uncertain whether those with alcohol dependence have an increased rate of crashes in the absence of raised blood alcohol levels, perhaps because, as this rarely occurs, it is methodologically difficult to study.

- Overall there is very good evidence that the crash rate in problem drinkers, ie those who have a history of convictions for drink/drive offences, is elevated.

- The determinants for progression from a 'problem drinker' with recurrent offences/crashes to an individual who develops long-term sequelae from alcohol dependence are not clear, although progression occurs in a significant proportion of convicted drink drivers.

- The relationships between alcohol misuse and dependence are not clear. There is evidence of a 'hardcore' group of alcohol-using repeat offenders, but they appear to represent one part of a spectrum of alcohol use, which includes a variety of traits leading to misuse and/or dependency.[3]

- In the driving population as a whole there is a well documented correlation between blood/breath alcohol levels and crash risk. There is no clear threshold below which impairment does not occur.

- The impairing effects of medications with psychoactive or sedating effects and non-prescribed drugs such as cannabis interact with those of alcohol to produce more severe impairment than would be the case from either acting alone.

- Both alcohol and drugs will increase the impairing effects of sleepiness in both those deprived of sleep and in those with sleep disorders.

The pharmacological effects and their timescale vary widely among different drugs and different methods of intake. Drug intake by the intravenous or inhaled routes has a much more immediate impact on impairment than more slowly absorbed routes such as ingestion. The use of multiple agents and their association with other mental health problems, in addition to dependence and misuse, or with criminal activities, also make for difficulties in determining the realities of their effects on driving.

The persistence of some commonly measured metabolites of cannabis, long after the impairing effects of the transient active metabolite have ceased, limits the use of biochemical methods to assess risk from the most commonly used non-therapeutic product.

For some agents such as benzodiazepines, initial prescription use can lead to subsequent dependency and this creates problems in defining whether the use is therapeutic or not. As with prescribed use, when used non-therapeutically these agents will severely impair driving.

Methadone, used as therapy for other opiate addiction, is itself impairing, and users may themselves overdose or combine it with other opiates or with drugs from other classes.

Evidence – non-therapeutic drugs

- Some substances are also used therapeutically (see p. 105).

- Effects are substance-specific. However, multiple drug use is common and may include all classes of drug as well as alcohol.

- Because of the illegality of drug use in most jurisdictions, there are limitations to the scope for carrying out experimental investigations, and self-reports of drug use are likely to be inaccurate.

- *Cannabis* impairs driving, but unlike other drugs the user is relatively aware of the impairment and in some cases can choose to compensate for it.

- *Opiates*. Those on methadone maintenance programmes, as well as a wide range of other potentially impairing problems, show excess levels of cognitive impairment.[4] However, the reality of unsafe driving has been questioned.[5]

- *Stimulants* can appear to enhance some of the skills needed in driving, such as reaction time, but evidence suggests an overall detrimental effect due to inappropriate reactions to events on the road.

- Evidence is lacking on the effect of *hallucinogenic drugs* on driving. The psychosis-like effects and visual distortions produced by hallucinogens would be expected to seriously impair capacity to drive.

Clinical assessment and advice

The DVLA lists criteria for:[6]

- *Alcohol misuse* – 'a state which, because of consumption of alcohol, causes disturbance of behaviour, related disease or other consequences, likely to cause the patient, their family or society harm now or in the future, and which may or may not be associated with dependency'.

- *Alcohol dependency* – 'a cluster of behavioural, cognitive and physiological phenomena that develop after repeated alcohol use and which include a strong desire to take alcohol, difficulties in controlling its use, persistence in its use despite harmful consequences, with

evidence of increased tolerance and sometimes a physical withdrawal state'. Indicators may include a history of withdrawal symptoms, of tolerance, of detoxification(s) and/or alcohol-related fits (see p. 130).

- *Alcohol-related disorders*, eg hepatic cirrhosis with neuropsychiatric impairment, psychosis.

- *Persistent use of or dependency on*:
  —cannabis, amphetamines, Ecstasy and other psychoactive substances, including LSD and hallucinogens
  —heroin, morphine, methadone, cocaine
  —benzodiazepines.

- *Methadone maintenance therapy*.

- Seizures associated with drug misuse/dependency (see p. 130).

These standards show the extent to which the assessment of fitness to drive in those who misuse or are dependent on alcohol or drugs differs from that needed for other conditions, where behavioural factors are not so dominant. For drugs the position is further complicated by their illegality. This means that the legal sanctions against possession or dealing have to be distinguished from those that relate to road safety. In particular, few of those who are dependent manage to separate use and driving so that their driving performance is not impaired by acute intoxication.

Few of those with notifiable problems are likely themselves to disclose them to the DVLA. Those in a clinical relationship who are trying to help the patient deal with the condition may find that, while the threat of loss of driving licence may be an incentive to follow advice, taking action to notify the DVLA because the patient has not done so can endanger the therapeutic relationship. It is good practice to inform patients of the risks and advise them to notify the DVLA, recording that this advice has been given. If there is persistent disregard of this advice in the presence of a known continuing risk, then the clinician may need to tell the patient that they will have to inform the DVLA (see p. 36). Agreeing with the patient that a second opinion is needed may be one solution.

The penalties for a conviction for driving while under the influence of drink or drugs should be brought to the attention of the patient. These are:

- minimum disqualification of one year
- fine of up to £5000
- up to six months in prison.

Attending a drink-driver rehabilitation course offered by the court at the time of sentencing for an alcohol-related offence shortens the period of exclusion from driving by three months when the disqualification is for the minimum of one year and up to 25% of the disqualification, at the court's discretion, for longer periods of disqualification.

The statutory High-Risk Offender Scheme provides a rather different regimen for those who have been disqualified:

- from driving with over 2.5 times the legal limit for alcohol
- for failing to provide, without reasonable excuse, a sample
- twice within 10 years for exceeding the legal limit.

At the end of their disqualification, but before a licence is again granted, they have to undergo (at their own expense) an independent medical examination by one of the doctors franchised by the DVLA to perform them. This includes clinical and biochemical assessments

looking for continuing risk factors and for effects of alcohol. A licence will not be issued if there are indications of a continuing problem.

Those in drug rehabilitation programmes need to meet the following criteria before re-licensing will be considered:

- rehabilitation in a consultant-led unit
- one year without the use of illicit drugs
- randomized drug testing used on participants
- supervised oral maintenance medication, or injected depot preparations given at the clinic.

References

1. Royal Society for the Prevention of Accidents. *Drinking and Driving Policy Paper*. Royal Society for the Prevention of Accidents, 2005. www.search.atomz.com/search/?sp-q=drinking+and+driving&sp-k=Road+Safety&submit=Go&sp-a=sp100314bd&sp-p=all&sp-f=ISO-8859-1

2. Charlton J, *et al. Influence of Chronic Illness on Crash Involvement of Motor Vehicle Drivers*. Report No. 213. Accident Research Centre, Monash University, 2004: 18–34. www.monash.edu.au/muarc/reports/muarc213.pdf

3. Chamberlain E, Solomon R. The tooth fairy, Santa Claus, and the hard core drinking driver. *Injury Prev* 2001; **7**: 272–275.

4. Darke S, Sims J, McDonald S, Wickes W. Cognitive impairment among methadone maintenance patients. *Addiction* 2000; **95**: 687-695.

5. Zachny JP. Should people taking opioids for medical reasons be allowed to work and drive? *Addiction* 1996; **91**: 1581–1584.

6. *At A Glance Guide*. Swansea: DVLA. www.dvla.gov.uk/at_a_glance/ch5_drugandalcohol.htm

SECTION 4: IMPAIRMENT OF MOVEMENT

Most injuries and the majority of surgical procedures limit an individual's ability to drive because of movement that is limited by pain, weakness or inflexibility. The exceptions are situations where other risks such as cognitive impairment, seizure, cardiac event or visual limitations are associated with the injury or surgery.

- Range, strength, precision and stamina of movements across joints can all be reduced.
- Reduction can be absolute or as a consequence of pain beyond certain limits. The latter will often lead to self-limitation of movement to avoid the pain.
- Pathology may be in the soft tissues, joints, bones, muscles, ligaments or tendons. It is also frequently a consequence of neurological disease that reduces the control of muscle movement.
- Abnormal muscular movements, such as jerking, writhing and severe tremors can all impair car control.
- Many forms of surgery and trauma limit driving, at least temporarily, because of interference with movement.
- The limitations from permanent limb and some other movement disabilities can be mitigated by adaptations to vehicles (see p. 49).

Variations in vehicle design, and hence choice of car, can play an important part in minimizing the effects of some types of musculoskeletal impairment.

- Good mirrors can provide rear vision if neck movements are limited.
- Automatic transmission will reduce the need for left-foot control and limit the need for the left arm to change gear.
- Power steering will reduce the demands for trunk, shoulder and arm strength.
- Power-assisted braking will reduce the need for forceful action by the right foot.
- A high seating position will be more accessible and comfortable for many drivers (and passengers) with limited strength or flexibility.
- Wide doors and low sills will aid entry and exit.
- Driving from a wheelchair may be feasible in a specially converted vehicle with the appropriate safety features.

15. Injury, surgery and musculoskeletal conditions

Impairment and risk
Clinical assessment and advice

Impairment and risk

The vast majority of injuries, if they impair driving, will do so primarily because of limitations to movement or other aspects of motor function. The exceptions are:

- *Injuries directly affecting sense organs*, especially vision (see p. 69). In addition to direct effects on the eye, musculoskeletal problems that limit neck mobility may also interfere with the recognition of visual cues to danger, especially where they are at the limits of the functional field of view gained by movements of the head as well as the eyes.

- *Head injuries* leading to changes in cognitive performance and in other facets of brain function (see p. 99).

The post-operative course from most forms of surgical intervention is also usually determined by recovery of motor function and any pain-related limitations. There are, however, other specific limitations from some forms of surgery: cardiac – cardiac event and cognitive impairment (see p. 136); eye – vision standards and prognosis (see p. 69; intracranial – seizure and residual impairment (see p. 129); hepatic – cognition (see p. 83).

The functional limitations to driving from musculoskeletal disease share many features with injuries but are either characterized by progressive limitations, as in the development of osteoarthritis, or by exacerbations and remissions, as in rheumatoid arthritis. Many musculoskeletal pain syndromes, such as those

that affect the neck or back, can be considered in very much the same way as injuries in terms of their effects on driving.

Evidence – musculoskeletal disease

- A number of studies of older drivers show an increased crash risk in those with limited ranges of movements in their limbs and neck.[1]

Impairment, usually cognitive, may occur from medication use, from the residual effects of anaesthetics used for surgery and for resetting fractures, and in particular from the prolonged use of analgesics for pain control.

The timeline after injury or surgery will normally consist of:

- An initial period when there is both loss of function and pain. There may also be general debilitation and loss of capacity to undertake cognitively demanding tasks at this time.

- A variable time when either pain has gone or it is only provoked by specific movements but there is not full motor function. Movement may be encouraged for some conditions, such as back pain, but artificially limited for others, such as fractures, to aid the healing process. There may be some loss of stamina, not least because of the tiring effects of having to live within the limitations of pain-restricted movements and of their disturbing effects on the length and quality of sleep.

- Concurrent with this there is often adaptation in posture and movement that enables the individual to increase their range of movements and pain-free tasks. This may be assisted by formal or informal rehabilitation activities.

- An end state which is, in most cases, full recovery but where there may still be some long-term or permanent motor limitations.

Similar, although not so clearly time-bound, deficits occur with musculoskeletal conditions.

After injuries and surgery, apart from those such as head injury or cardiac surgery where there could be an excess risk of sudden incapacity, it is likely to be the person's immediate present state that determines whether they can drive safely. Safety will be determined not just by the requirements of normal driving, but also by the need to use additional strength or speed of action in pre-accident conditions, such as the application of immediate hard pressure to the brake pedal during an emergency stop, while being aware of the position of other road users. An indication that such responses would be inhibited, eg by pain or fear of pain after abdominal surgery, hernia repair or leg injury, can be expected both to increase the risk and to impair recovery should emergency action be taken with damage to the process of healing.

There are no valid studies looking at driving risk after injuries or surgery, nor are there data linked to licensing, because notification to the licensing authority is not normally required. It would be difficult to design a sound study to investigate the effects on driving of performance limited by pain and stamina because of the transient and variable pattern of impairment. Such studies would be severely confounded by decisions taken by the driver or advice given by health professionals on how much to limit driving in the short term after surgery or injury.

Cognitive impairment may persist for a period after cardiac surgery where cardiopulmonary bypass is used during the operation. Some forms of hepatic surgery where the liver is bypassed permanently as part of the procedure have been shown to lead to measurable cognitive impairment. There are no data on driving risk.

The effects of chronic longer-term musculoskeletal diseases on driving have been investigated, especially in older drivers. There is no evidence of excess risk, although it is likely that most drivers will modify their driving patterns to take account of any limitation, especially those that lead to pain or excessive fatigue.

Damage to neuromuscular control and function is often part of wider neurological disease processes, with a few exceptions such as motor neurone disease where it is limited to muscular control. There is no specific information on driving risk.

In the case of long-term or stable disability, modifications to the vehicle or to driving patterns can play an important part in maintaining mobility without excess risk. There is no evidence on the effects of informal vehicle choice or modification to accident risks, but there are good indications that those who have vehicle modifications to cope with disabilities following an assessment of needs have an accident rate comparable with that of other drivers.

Clinical assessment and advice

The key points to consider are:

- present state of the patient and their likely progress
- whether any current or likely future limitations on strength or movement may interfere with normal driving or prevent emergency actions
- whether limitation of movement from pain, or fear of pain, impairs normal driving or may inhibit essential emergency actions
- whether the individual is debilitated by their condition such that cognition or stamina is impaired
- whether any devices used, such as casts on limbs or neck collars, will limit safe driving
- effects of any medication on driving performance.

The experience the individual has of their condition and their self-awareness of any difficulties in driving will both play a major part in deciding on the advice to be given. For example, where driving is a requirement for work, then the ability to drive at set times of the day, often first thing in the morning when any stiffness is usually at its greatest, may have to be considered.

The potential for inhibition of emergency actions because of fear of pain is also difficult to assess in the clinical setting. A number of the available guidelines about how long to wait before returning to driving after surgery or treatment for trauma have their origins in concern about this aspect. Most available guidelines on how long to wait before returning to driving after surgery or treatment for trauma are consensus documents based on the experience of those who regularly perform certain procedures.

Return to driving after surgical procedures

When giving advice, the health professional needs to take into account any co-morbidity from other impairing conditions, as well as the effects of the surgery.

- In all cases, the *effects of anaesthesia, pain control or other impairing medication and discomfort from sutures* should no longer be present. Following general anaesthesia, drivers should be advised not to drive at least for the rest of the day. A normal pattern of sleeping and eating should have returned. There should not be any consequential risks of impairment or incapacity, eg from removal of endocrine tissue or from a new stoma.

- *Abdomen, back and chest*. Resume driving after demonstrating that the necessary strength, range of non-pain-limited motion and stamina are present.

- *Cardiac* (see p. 136).

- *Intracranial* (see p. 129).

- *Renal transplant* – off for four weeks.[2]

- *Orthopaedic procedures* will usually directly affect the limbs and may require immobilization or a period without weight bearing. Because the limbs are essential for car control, some authorities have made specific recommendations.[3]

- *Amputation*. Car adaptation is normally required prior to return to driving.

- *Anterior cruciate ligament*. Four weeks off for either leg, unless the patient's car has automatic transmission and surgery is to the left leg, then return when comfortable to do so.

- *Limb fractures involving splints or casts*. No restriction unless splint/cast interferes with driving. If it does, the patient should stop driving until the cast has been removed and their strength and range of motion have returned.

- *Rotator cuff repair* – open or arthroscopic. Off for four to six weeks if car has power steering, longer if not.

- *Shoulder reconstruction* – off for four to six weeks if car has power steering, longer if not.

- *Total hip replacement* – off for four weeks. If their car has automatic transmission, the patient may re-start driving when comfortable to do so if the surgery has been to the left hip. The patient needs to take special care when transferring to vehicles, so that hip flexion greater than 90° is avoided. Care is also needed, as reaction times in the limb may be slowed for up to eight weeks.

- *Total knee arthroplasty* – off for 3–4 weeks. If car has automatic transmission, may re-start driving when comfortable to do so if they have had surgery to the left knee. Care is also needed, as the reaction times in the limb may be slowed for up to eight weeks.

Care is needed about transfers in and out of cars when patients are travelling as passengers after orthopaedic surgery. It is important that seat belts are correctly worn even in the presence of casts, splints or healing incisions.

Advice based on fixed times off driving after surgery may be useful and defensible in deciding on time away from work if driving to or at work is essential. However, there is considerable individual variability, with some of 'the tail of disability' having psychosocial components such as attitudes to work or the search for blame and compensation for an injury. In those for whom driving is part of their work, any other demands, such as loading or unloading goods or equipment or securing loads, also need to be considered.

In those with recent injuries or surgery, an informal self-assessment of performance while stationary and then on quiet roads, where the full range of driving movements is required for steering, gear change and rear vision, can be useful.[4] It should include a trial emergency stop. Action may be based on the individual's views or follow a feedback session with the health professional. If this approach is suggested, then it is usually wise to recommend that journeys are initially fairly short, with progressive extension. This is to avoid the effects of longer-term postural or fatigue problems until their likely severity has been assessed closer to home.

Where there are continuing residual effects from surgery or injury, or where there are long-term musculoskeletal problems, then ways in which the driving task can be modified to fit the vehicle around the individual's capabilities have to be considered.[5]

Specific musculoskeletal problems

The following may pose particular problems for driving:

- *Foot abnormalities* that limit flexion or extension of the ankle or contact with foot pedals (eg ankle joint limitations, bunions, hammer toes, calluses, overgrown toe nails). These should be treated where possible and, if this is not possible, use of vehicle adaptations with training in their use should be considered. There is some evidence that associates structural and functional foot abnormalities, and also complaints of cold feet and legs, with higher crash and traffic incident rates.[6]
- *Limitations of cervical movement* reducing the effective range of vision. Training in mirror use or fitting additional rear-view aids should be considered.

- *Severe limitations or deformities of thoracic or lumbar spine.* Specially designed car seating may be needed, possibly with modifications to the position of controls or to mirrors. Driving should cease if there are unstabilized or painful spinal conditions that interfere with car control.
- Some evidence indicates that older drivers with a history of *back pain* and those with a history of *bursitis* have both elevated crash and traffic incident risks.[7]
- *Loss of extremities and use of prostheses.* Special adaptations will be needed. Lower-limb prostheses will not have the required sensory feedback for pedal controls, and hand controls are needed.

Although not strictly a musculoskeletal problem, deep vein thrombosis can have an impairing effect on leg mobility. Driving can re-commence when there is adequate dorsiflexion of the ankle to enable pedal control. Breaks to mobilize the limb should be taken at frequent intervals on long journeys, whether the patient is driving or travelling as a passenger.

Assessment of the present state of neuromuscular control, in the absence of other impairments, will determine current capability for driving. Prognosis will be a guide to future needs, expectations and any required adaptations.

- The known progression of *motor neurone disease* should signal early recourse to a suitably adapted vehicle or to alternative mobility arrangements.
- The exacerbations and remissions of *multiple sclerosis* will indicate the need for the driver to be able to decide on their day-to-day capacity for safe car control.
- The pattern of an individual's recovery from *stroke* or *peripheral neuropathic disabilities* will help to determine future needs for vehicle adaptation or alternative mobility aids.

Many drivers will make modifications themselves, but some prompting may be needed.

- Can journey patterns be changed to avoid, for example, long periods at the wheel or reversing to park?

- Can simple and safe additions to an existing vehicle be made, eg use of a back support, larger rear-view mirrors?

- Should the vehicle be changed now or later to one with a more appropriate specification – larger doors, more upright seating, automatic transmission, lighter steering, rear-load area without high sill?

- Is an expert assessment needed, including the scope for engineering modifications to a vehicle (see p. 49)?

- Is the present state or prognosis such that driving may be in jeopardy in future? If so, the individual may need to consider where to live to be less car dependent or anticipate any other consequences for their working or domestic life.

- Could the management of their condition be adjusted to make driving safer or less limited – by careful choice of medication for effectiveness without sedation, surgical treatment of pain-limited joints, choice of prosthesis in amputees?

The risks of sudden incapacity or of cognitive impairment after a few forms of surgery/injury also need to be considered, and it is these rather than the normal pattern of recovery that require a decision on whether to continue to license a driver.

Where engineering modifications to a car are made, drivers of such vehicles are issued with a special class of licence (see p. 49).

References

1. *Safe Mobility for Older Drivers. IA2(a) Physical Performance Deficits*. Washington, DC: National Highway Transportation Safety Administration, 2000: 29–31. www.nhtsa.dot.gov/people/injury/olddrive/safe/ safe-toc.htm

2. *Physician's Guide to Assessing and Counseling Older Drivers*. Washington, DC: National Highway Transportation Safety Administration, 2003, Chapter 9, Section 10: 1. www.nhtsa.dot.gov/people/injury/ olddrive/OlderDriversBook/pages/Ch9-Section10.html

3. ibid: Section 8: 2–4. www.nhtsa.dot.gov/people/injury/ olddrive/OlderDriversBook/pages/Ch9-Section8.html

4. Nunez VA, Giddins GEB. 'Doctor, when can I drive?': an update on the medico-legal aspects of driving following an injury or operation. *Injury* 2004; **35**: 888–890

5. Driving with arthritis. www.arc.org.uk/about_arth/booklets/6011/6011.htm

6. *Safe Mobility for Older Drivers. IA1(e) Foot Abnormalities, (h) Feet or Legs Cold on Exposure to Cold*. Washington, DC: National Highway Transportation Safety Administration, 2000: 12–13 and 17–18. www.nhtsa.dot.gov/people/ injury/olddrive/safe/safe-toc.htm

7. ibid. *(i) Bursitis, (l) Back pain*: 18–19 and 21.

SECTION 5: SUDDEN INCAPACITY

Loss of consciousness or an altered state of awareness is a self-evident risk if it occurs while an individual is driving and comes on too quickly to allow them to stop the vehicle safely.

- There may be circumstances where an increased risk of loss or alteration of consciousness can be anticipated, eg from seizures after a severe head injury or syncope as a consequence of some cardiac arrhythmias.

- There are many instances where a 'collapse' or sudden loss of consciousness is reported by a patient, but only with limited information about the antecedents to and clinical course of the event. Information of this sort is important in helping to identify the likely relevance of the event to driving, for deciding how to investigate and treat it, and for estimating the probability of a recurrence. In the absence of adequate information a precautionary approach may be indicated.

- When the probability of a recurrence is uncertain, the individual may need a period of observation to see if there is a regular pattern to events. During this time the individual should be advised to avoid tasks such as driving which could pose a risk to others in the event of a recurrence.

- If there are repeated events, or if a well-defined cause is found for a single event, treatments such as anti-epileptic medications for seizures or a cardiac pacemaker for an arrhythmia may be indicated.

The most important indicators of driving risk are the speed of onset of incapacity from the event and whether there are warning symptoms/signs which, if heeded, will enable the driver to abort the event or to immobilize the vehicle safely.

One UK study from 1983 does provide an indication of the relative importance of different causes of sudden incapacity at the time of the study, although the attribution of cause can often only be made on the balance of probabilities:[1]

- coronary heart attack – 10%
- stroke – 7%
- hypoglycaemia – 17%
- epilepsy – 50%.

Examples of warning symptoms/signs include the following:

- *Seizures* will sometimes be preceded by an aura, but if they are not then incapacitation can be instant. Seizures are generally unrelated to current external conditions, with rare exceptions such as photosensitive seizures caused by stroboscopic effects from lighting, or in the medium term the excess risk associated with some medications and with alcohol.

- By contrast *syncopal unconsciousness* is caused by cerebral anoxia. This can be triggered by posture, heat or emotion (neurogenic syncope), which all lead to reduced venous return to the heart. Here unconsciousness is not usually instantaneous. It is often preceded by air hunger, feelings of faintness and other symptoms. Cough syncope is also a result of reduced venous return, but the coughing fit itself can incapacitate prior to unconsciousness. Reduced cardiac output from deficiencies in pumping action, usually because of an arrhythmia, or from valve malfunction, will also lead to cerebral ischaemia, which can sometimes cause unconsciousness without prior warning (drop attack) (see p. 137).

- *Hypoglycaemia from insulin* – another expression of the brain being starved of nutrients – often has its own characteristic warning signs, which can include confusion and changes in behaviour. The pace of onset is such that if there are warning signs and they are acted on, unconsciousness can usually be avoided (see p. 143).

Because of the diversity and transience of such episodes of incapacity there is little scope for identifying their causal role in accidents or for investigating them using simulator studies. For certain defined categories of cause, such as specific cardiac arrhythmias and clinically confirmed first seizures, there are prognostic data on recurrence. However, in many cases the reason for the initial loss of consciousness or awareness is uncertain and there is no scope for using condition-specific recurrence data to predict future risk.[2]

Based on studies of seizure risk, initially from head injury and then in those with epilepsy, an increased incidence of sudden incapacity of less than 2% per year came into use as a benchmark for removal of restrictions on Group 2 driving, and less than 20% per year for Group 1. These benchmarks seem to have stood the test of time in terms of being a rational and acceptable set of criteria and so have subsequently been used as broad guides to the levels of tolerable risk from other causes of sudden incapacity (see p. 57).

References

1. Taylor JF. Epilepsy and other causes of collapse at the wheel. In: Godwin Austin RB, Espir MLE, eds. *Driving and Epilepsy – and Other Causes of Impaired Consciousness.* Royal Society of Medicine International Congress and Symposium Series No. 60. London: Academic Press/Royal Society of Medicine, 1983.

2. Task Force on Syncope, European Society of Cardiology. Part 1. The initial evaluation of patients with syncope. *Europace* 2001; **3**: 253–260.

16. Loss of consciousness or altered awareness

Assessment of causation and risks

Assessment of causation and risks

The key to assessing the risks while driving is determining the probable cause of the event. Events can be categorized into one of five types:[1]

1. *Simple faint* – definite provocational factors, with associated prodromal symptoms that are unlikely to occur while the individual is sitting or lying. It is benign in nature. If faints are recurrent, confirmation is needed that each event is associated with a provoking situation, prodromal symptoms and a posture other than sitting. If in doubt proceed to type 3. No restrictions on driving need be advised.

2. *Loss of consciousness/loss of or altered awareness is likely to be an unexplained syncope* and has a low risk of recurrence if:
    —there is no abnormality of the cardiovascular system
    —the neurological examination is normal
    —the ECG shows no relevant abnormality.

3. *Loss of consciousness/altered awareness is likely to be an unexplained syncope* but has a high risk of recurrence if there is one or more of:
    —abnormal ECG
    —clinical evidence of structural heart disease
    —syncope causing injury, occurring at the wheel or while sitting or lying
    —more than one episode in the last six months.

Further investigations such as ambulatory ECG (24 hour), echocardiography and exercise testing may be indicated after a specialist opinion has been sought.

4. *Unwitnessed (presumed) loss of consciousness/altered awareness with seizure markers*. This category is for those where there is a strong clinical suspicion of epilepsy but no definite evidence. The seizure markers act as indicators and are not absolutes:
    —unconsciousness for more than five minutes
    —amnesia greater than five minutes
    —injury
    —tongue biting, especially of the side
    —incontinence, but this may also occur in syncope
    —remaining conscious but with confused behaviour
    —headache post attack.

5. *Loss of consciousness/altered awareness with no clinical pointers*. This category will have had neurological and cardiological opinion and investigations but with no abnormality detected.

Decisions on categories 3–5 should be taken by the licensing authority. A period without driving to ensure that there is no early recurrence will normally be required. This will be longer if a seizure was the presumed cause. In category 3 the period may be shortened if a cause has been found and is treated. In all cases the period off driving will be longer for drivers of large vehicles.

If the event is diagnosed from observation by witnesses or clinical review as a first seizure or a solitary fit, then different considerations apply (see p. 130). Similarly a different approach is needed if an underlying cardiac malfunction is identified (see Chapter 19).

Cough syncope presents a particular set of risks, as the syncope can be provoked in a sitting position and the individual is usually at least partially incapacitated by the coughing spasm. Hence they are unable to immobilize the vehicle safely before loss of consciousness.[2] As the underlying cause of the condition is usually chronic lung disease, it is likely that the risk of provocation will remain present. The DVLA should be informed. A period of freedom from attacks will be needed before return to driving, and this may be long term or indefinite in those with chronic lung disease who drive

large vehicles. If it can be shown that asystole was the response to the coughing spasm and this can be corrected with a pacemaker, an earlier return to driving may be possible.[3]

The assessment of, advice to and notification requirements for persons with loss of consciousness, seizures and epilepsy are summarized in Table 16.1.

Table 16.1
Assessment, advice and notification – loss of consciousness, seizures and epilepsy.

Condition	Clinician assessment specific to driving	Recommendations to driver	Notification to the DVLA
Simple faint	Confirm markers: • prodrome • posture • provocation	Report any future events	No
Loss of consciousness – low-recurrence risk	Confirm absence of neurological or cardiac risk factors	Stop driving Group 1 – 4 weeks Group 2 – 3 months	No No
Loss of consciousness – high risk of recurrence	Presence of neurological or cardiac risk factors	Stop driving Group 1 – 4 weeks if cause found, 6 months if no cause found Group 2 – 3 months if cause found, 1 year if no cause found	No Yes Yes
Loss of consciousness with seizure markers	Presence of seizure markers	Stop driving	Yes
Loss of consciousness – no clinical pointers	Potential for seizure – lack of observer, memory, etc	Stop driving	Yes
Cough syncope	Confirm link to coughing and exclude other causes	Stop driving	Yes
Epilepsy	Check if secure new diagnosis or recurrence	Stop driving	Yes
First seizure	Confirm it is first event	Stop driving	Yes
Withdrawal of anti-epileptic medication	Check absence of seizures during process	Group 1 – stop for 6 months. Then restart if no further seizures Group 2 – not applicable	No
Provoked seizure (see p. 130)	Confirm presence of provocation and absence of prior seizures	Stop driving	Yes
Seizure associated with alcohol or non-medicinal drugs	Confirm association with alcohol or drug use	Stop driving	Yes

References

1. Neurological conditions. In: *At A Glance Guide*. Swansea: DVLA. www.dvla.gov.uk/at_a_glance/ch1_neurological.htm

2. McCorry DJ, Chadwick DW. Cough syncope in heavy goods vehicle drivers. *Q J Med* 2004; **97**: 631–632.

3. Choi YS, *et al*. Cough syncope caused by sinus arrest in a patient with sick sinus syndrome. *Pacing Clin Electrophysiol* 1989; **12**: 883–886.

17. Seizures and epilepsy

Impairment and risk
Clinical assessment and advice

Impairment and risk

Epilepsy is one of the few specific medical conditions where diagnosis leads to prohibition of driving under primary legislation. An increased risk of seizures can arise in a number of situations including, among others:

- after a head injury
- following intracranial surgery
- following a stroke
- with a cancer where secondary deposits in the brain are likely
- as a continuing trait in an individual with a previous history of epilepsy
- during withdrawal of anti-epileptic medication
- with some medications
- associated with high intake of alcohol or other non-therapeutic drug use or during a period of withdrawal from use.

The diagnosis of seizure is essentially a clinical one based on a description of symptoms and an eyewitness account of the event. Making such a diagnosis can be difficult, especially where the event has not happened before and where there are no identifiable predisposing factors.[1–3] There may be many reasons why the event is not fully disclosed, and fear of being unable to drive is one. The clinical presentation of a seizure varies widely, and often, but not always, follows a constant pattern in an individual if it recurs.

Evidence – risks from seizure[2]

- It is methodologically difficult to perform studies: those with poorly controlled epilepsy are normally excluded from driving, there are big personal incentives not to declare a seizure,[4] and the immediate antecedents of a crash will only rarely be witnessed.

- The majority of studies have shown increased crash risk in those with epilepsy, but the level of excess varies widely among studies and may reflect demographic variables and distances travelled.

- A long period since the last seizure seems to be the best predictor of lack of excess risk. A number of large population studies have been the source of estimates of future risk. While there is some evidence of reductions in recurrence rates from better therapy of epilepsy and from better treatment of head injuries and other predisposing factors, there are insufficient recent data to improve the current estimates.[5]

- Cessation of anti-epilepsy medication is associated with a period when there is an increase in risk.

- The relative risks from different forms of seizure disorder have not been well investigated. Some persistent patterns, such as seizures showing a well-established pattern of only occurring during sleep, may indicate a low level of risk while driving. (Narcolepsy, which is predominantly a condition leading to sudden sleep, is considered with other sleep disorders in Chapter 21.)

- People who have failed to declare their epilepsy do have crashes attributable to seizures at the wheel. Crashes attributable to a seizure in those who have notified and been re-licensed after the required seizure-free period are very rare. Both these statements are based on police accident reports rather than rigorous studies.

Functional impairment from seizures can vary widely.[6] But most of the forms of altered consciousness that arise will impair driving. For this reason propensity to seizures of any sort, except where their timing is such that they never happen at times when driving takes place, may be seen as a risk, although there are variations in the approaches of different national licensing bodies to forms of seizure which are not incapacitating. The sedating effects of some anti-epilepsy medications also need to be considered.

Where there are known provoking factors such as stroboscopic lighting, then avoidance may be possible. Where seizures are an uncommon side effect of a medication, then a personal risk assessment may be possible and may form the basis for advice. However, where seizures are linked to lifestyle factors, such as alcohol misuse, recurrence is in practice frequent. It is not possible to identify the cause of a single seizure at a time when there could have been provocation. The provoking agent may have been a sole and sufficient cause; it may have unmasked an underlying excess risk or it may have simply been coincidental to the event.

Seizure risk is one of the few examples of the use of the results from large studies of populations either at risk of epilepsy from head injury or with idiopathic epilepsy to predict the likely seizure risk for an individual, and then to use this to decide on fitness to drive. The cut-off levels have been developed pragmatically, first using head injury data, where the nature and severity of the trauma are a major determinant of risk, and then extending these to intracranial surgery and later to epilepsy in general as comparable results have become available.[7] Level of risk of a seizure in the next year (for head injury) or a recurrent seizure in the next year (for idiopathic epilepsy) is determined by the time since the last seizure. If anti-epileptic medication is stopped or reduced, there is a period of increased risk over the next few months,[8] but, in the absence of a recurrence during this period, the risk then follows a downward curve. Despite some statistical controversy about the actual levels of risk, especially the way in which to statistically handle those who do have a subsequent seizure and then re-enter the population being studied, this form of risk stratification has enabled a rationale for standards for the recurrence of sudden incapacitating events to be developed. Two widely used risk thresholds are:[9]

- *Less than 20% risk of seizure in the next year.* This level of risk is found after one year without a seizure. The use of medication does not affect the risk, as the probability of recurrence after one year free of seizures is the same in groups where no medication has been taken and in groups complying with the use of anti-epilepsy medication.

- *Less than 2% risk of seizure in the next year.* This expected rate of recurrence is not reached until 10 years free from seizures have passed, without the use of anti-epilepsy medication at any time during this period.

Clinical assessment and advice

The risk of sudden incapacitation from a seizure, whatever the cause, will always have implications for driving. Because, in legal terms, epilepsy is defined in UK regulation as a 'relevant disability', notification by the driver to the DVLA is always required. The DVLA will then use risk-based criteria to decide how long the individual needs to stop driving for and to specify any other conditions that may apply. The current risk criteria are those noted above: one year seizure-free on no medication or complying with medication use for a car (Group 1) driver; 10 years without a seizure and not on any anti-epileptic medication for a large vehicle (Group 2) driver. The same 20% per annum and 2% per annum criteria form the basis for the assessment of those who have had head injuries or intracranial surgery.

A single seizure, while not covered by the epilepsy regulations, also needs notification to the DVLA and a period away from driving to confirm that it is not the first of a recurring trait.

Similarly, some seizures where there appears to be provocation may be considered by the DVLA on an individual basis, especially in the following circumstances:[10]

- eclamptic
- reflex anoxic (syncope with convulsions and not a form of epilepsy)
- within seconds of a head injury (concussive convulsions and not a form of epilepsy)
- within a week of a head injury if there are no other signs suggesting serious damage
- within 24 hours of a stroke/transient ischaemic attack
- during or within 24 hours of intracranial surgery.

Because of these well-specified requirements and the active involvement of the DVLA in all decision-taking, the prime roles of the clinician are to:

- Ensure that the diagnosis is correctly made, either in terms of previous loss of, or alteration to, consciousness and whether an epileptiform seizure was responsible.
- Recognize any factors that may increase the liability to seizures, such as cranial trauma, either from injury or surgery (see p. 99), or epileptogenic medication, drug or alcohol use (see Chapter 14), or external stimuli such as stroboscopic lighting.
- Check compliance with medication use and advise of any side effects from anti-epileptic medication that could impair driving.
- Warn the driver of the risks of non-compliance both as regards accidents and in relation to the law and their insurance cover.
- If it is decided to withdraw medication or to modify it, ensure that the driver is aware that this may result in a period of driving cessation.[10]
- Inform drivers of their personal obligation

to notify the DVLA, check that this has been done and, where needed, follow up on any non-compliance.

- Ensure that, where treatment of injury, surgery or medication may increase seizure risk, patients are fully aware of this and have the opportunity to discuss its implications where feasible.
- Give interim recommendations prior to the DVLA advising on licensing status. Where the condition is such that it would not meet the current DVLA fitness standards, then cessation of driving should be recommended.
- Counsel the driver on the potential risks to self and others of continuing to drive and, based on DVLA guidelines or on the decision taken by the DVLA, help with re-adaptation during any period when driving is not permitted.
- Provide any additional information that the DVLA may request to assist with reaching a fair decision on a driver.

References

1. Charlton J, et al. *Influence of Chronic Illness on Crash Involvement of Motor Vehicle Drivers*. Report No. 213. Accident Research Centre, Monash University, 2004: 183–194. www.monash.edu.au/muarc/reports/muarc213.pdf

2. Dobbs BM. *Medical Conditions and Driving: A Review of the Literature 1960–2000*. DOT HS 809 690. Washington, DC: National Highway Transportation Safety Administration, 2005: 59–61. www.nhtsa.dot.gov/people/injury/research/MedicalConditions_Driving.pdf

3. *Safe Mobility for Older Drivers. IA1(k) Seizure Disorders*. Washington, DC: National Highways Transportation Safety Administration, 2000: 19–21. www.nhtsa.dot.gov/people/injury/olddrive/safe/safe-toc.htm

4. Dalrymple J, Appleby J. Cross sectional study of reporting epileptic seizures to general practitioners. *BMJ* 2000; **320**: 94–97.

5. *Epilepsy and Driving in Europe*. Report of Medical Working Group, EU Driver Licensing Committee, 2005. www.europa.eu.int/comm/transport/home/drivinglicence/fitnesstodrive/index_en.htm

6. Charlton J, et al. *Influence of Chronic Illness on Crash Involvement of Motor Vehicle Drivers*. Report No. 213. Accident Research Centre, Monash University, 2004: 180–185. www.monash.edu.au/muarc/reports/muarc213.pdf

7. Medical Research Council Anti-Epileptic Drug Withdrawal

Study Group. Prognostic index of the recurrence of seizures after remission of epilepsy. *BMJ* 1993; **306**: 1374–1378.

8. Medical Research Council Anti-Epileptic Drug Withdrawal Study Group. Randomised study of anti-epileptic drug withdrawal in patients in remission. *Lancet* 1991; **337**: 1175–1180.

9. Jennett B. Epilepsy and neurological disorders. In: Taylor J, Ed. *Medical Aspects of Fitness to Driver* 5th edn. Medical Commission on Accident Prevention, 1995: 78–82.

10. Neurological conditions. *At A Glance Guide*. Swansea: DVLA. www.dvla.gov.uk/at_a_glance/ ch1_neurological.htm

18. Tumours and cancers

**Impairment and risk
Clinical assessment and advice**

Impairment and risk

The nature of impairment from tumours and other malignant conditions is so variable that only the features regularly relevant to driving are reviewed here.

Probably the most serious risk is of a seizure as a result of a primary or secondary intracranial tumour. There are no data specific to driving, but a raised incidence of seizures from primary brain tumours, both as a presenting symptom and as a consequence of recurrence after treatment, is well recognized. In addition, in those tumours that commonly metastasize to the brain, such as lung cancer and melanoma, a seizure may be the first evidence of spread. Probability data for cerebral metastases and for seizures as a consequence are available.[1]

Intracranial tumours may also lead to a wide range of focal neurological deficits, as well as to less well localized effects on mental function. These can cause driving impairment or require vehicle modification to overcome persistent limitations in the individual's coordination or motor function following treatment.

Pituitary tumours, because of their location, may press on the optic chiasma and present with or cause defects in the field of vision (see p. 72).

- Tumours at other than intracranial sites or likely to metastasize elsewhere do not present any consistent pattern of risk for driving.

- Pain or limitations on mobility after surgery can impair driving.
- The disease itself, as well as chemotherapy and radiotherapy, leads to debilitation.
- Strong analgesics and/or the pain that they are being used to treat can impair effective cognitive functioning (see p. 105).

Clinical assessment and advice

- *Cerebral tumours and known cerebral secondaries* – in most cases the decision is likely to be one for the licensing authority (see Table 12.1).

  However, for pituitary and benign infratentorial tumours the risks are low. In such cases drivers of both cars and large vehicles will usually be able to return to driving on recovery or after a short period off.

- *Cancers with a significant risk of metastasizing to the brain*: lung cancer is the most common example.

  —For car drivers no specific advice is required unless there are cerebral secondaries. If these are present, driving should cease and the patient should be advised to notify the DVLA.

  —For lung cancer in Group 2 drivers the DVLA should be notified and they may require a period off driving and brain scan evidence that no secondaries are present.

  —For other cancers where brain secondaries are a risk, drivers of large vehicles should be advised to notify the DVLA and may have a period of restriction.

- *Other tumours and their treatment* – advice on fitness to drive should form a part of wider discussions about future lifestyle and the impact of the illness. In particular, advice is needed on the likely ability of patients to drive themselves to and from debilitating sessions of therapy, as well as advice on the likely bar on driving if and when strong analgesics are required for pain relief. Guidance will need to be based on the site of the lesion and on the proposed approaches to treatment.

Reference

1. Evans S. Malignant disease. In: Rainford DJ, Gradwell DP, eds. *Aviation Medicine*. London: Hodder Arnold, 2006: 665–681.

19. Cardiovascular disease

Impairment and risk
Clinical assessment and advice

Impairment and risk

The most important safety-critical impairments are:

- recurrence of a cardiac event or the development of a new one that leads to sudden incapacity while driving
- episodic disorder of cardiac rhythm causing reduced cardiac output and resulting in syncope or impaired functioning
- more rarely, sudden major haemorrhage from a ruptured aneurysm.

Other relevant forms of impairment are:

- fatigue from the consequences of reduced circulatory performance
- cognitive impairment associated with heart failure, hypertension or bypass surgery
- anoxia secondary to vessel blockage, rupture or dissection affecting essential sensory or motor functions, eg vision, musculoskeletal function.

The functional consequences of impaired cerebral blood supply leading to stroke and transient ischaemic attack (TIA) are discussed as neurological conditions (see Chapter 12).

A range of vascular conditions can lead to sudden incapacity. In most cases this is a consequence of cerebral anoxia from reduced flow of oxygenated blood to the brain, sometimes termed cardiac syncope. Sudden onset of pain or other symptoms can severely impair driving ability, but they can also provide early warning of impending loss of

consciousness, especially when caused by an acute ischaemic event. A common feature of cerebral anoxia is that, while development is rapid, it is not usually instantaneous. There may be a period of 10–100 seconds when there is awareness of the event but not total incapacity. This may sometimes be sufficient to enable the driver to take action to mitigate crash risk by stopping and pulling their vehicle to one side of the road. Warning symptoms may be less reliable for severe reductions in cardiac output arising from ventricular arrhythmias and heart block. Where there is a less severe reduction in effective pumping, eg with sinus rhythm giving way to atrial fibrillation or flutter, incapacity may either develop over a longer period or be only partial.

Several forms of pathology can lead to sudden-onset cardiac events. By far the most common is atheromatous arterial disease, but others include abnormal foci for exciting cardiac muscle contraction, rheumatic valve disease and the cardiomyopathies. In addition, the use of implanted defibrillators to correct dangerous arrhythmias will also cause immediate subjective effects on activation, which may be incapacitating. The diffuse nature of atheromatous arterial disease means that the condition can present as several different forms of acute incapacity, including myocardial infarction, arrhythmias and stroke, as well as transient ischaemia affecting the heart muscle (causing angina), leg muscles (causing intermittent claudication) and cerebral blood flow (causing temporary ischaemic changes in function) (see p. 93).

Given these features, the key to assessing risk should be an estimate of the probability of such an episode in an individual. Unfortunately, while such sudden incapacity is important for driving, events of this sort are not routinely recorded in clinical practice, as in most cases there is full or partial recovery after an episode. Sudden incapacity, however, would pose a risk if the individual were at the wheel when it occurred. There are much more reliable data on recurrences leading to death or hospitalization.

Data, however, do show that the majority of collapses at the wheel are in those with a known history of heart disease and that this excess is highest soon after a previous cardiac event.[1]

Investigations have been undertaken to look for associations between cardiovascular disease as a whole, syncope, arrhythmias, coronary heart disease and road crashes. The results have not shown any clear links.

Evidence – cardiovascular disease and road safety[2,3]

- There is no consistent body of evidence that links cardiovascular disease as a whole or any of its specific forms to increased crash risk. A number of large population-based studies have been performed but their results are conflicting.
- One study of citations has shown that there is an increased rate of crashes in older drivers with cardiovascular disease. Following a special medical examination to determine continuing fitness to drive, the rate fell to the same as that of the general population in those who continued driving.
- No studies on driving performance have been reported.

Cardiovascular disease is a common cause of sudden death, and studies of death at the wheel indicate its importance. However, crashes attributable to it and resulting in damage to other vehicles or injury to other road users are uncommon.

Because of the uncertainties about prognosis and the rapidity of incapacity, it is not possible to develop criteria for cardiovascular disease that are precise and potentially related to driving risk, of the sort developed for seizure risks. However, the same 2% and 20% criteria are used for general guidance (see p. 57). The aviation industry has used a risk of cardiovascular fatality less than 1% in the next year as its basis for decisions on the fitness of commercial pilots, and the evidence used for this can also inform driving risk assessments.[4]

Evidence – sudden death at the wheel[5]

- Sudden death at the wheel is a rare event (<1–3.5% of crash records).
- Post-mortem data (14 studies) show that more than 80% of these drivers have cardiovascular disease and more than 70% show evidence of coronary artery disease. In one study more than 90% had cardiac hypertrophy.
- Injury to others was rare in early studies, but more recent investigations show an increase in passenger deaths – possibly as a consequence of increased road speeds or traffic density.
- Prodromal symptoms before the final journey had been reported to others by 25–40% of those dying.
- The only evidence on warning of event prior to incapacitation is indirect. One study showed that in only 2 of 44 deaths were there signs of braking prior to death. However, the most commonly noted site for an at-wheel fatality is in the car halted at the side of the road, suggesting some warning and a response to it.
- The role of the demands of driving in sudden events is uncertain. One study showed that, whilst there were no ECG changes while driving in those without cardiovascular disease, 17% of those with coronary artery disease showed significant changes.

Cardiac events (including recent myocardial infarction, unstable angina, recent cardiac surgical or percutaneous intervention)

The inherent limitations of studies to quantify the risk from immediate incapacitation mean that the major source of information used to predict risk while driving comes from the large morbidity and mortality studies on the prognosis of cardiovascular conditions and interventions. These cannot provide any information on absolute risk while driving, but they may enable the relative risk of different conditions and patterns of recovery to be stratified. As such studies are done over long time periods, the pattern of risk may relate to forms of disease or treatment that are no longer relevant. This is a particular problem where data on recurrence after medical and surgical interventions are used, as these change rapidly. In addition, diagnostic criteria may change, especially when new investigative methods, such as tropinin release as an indicator of heart muscle damage, are introduced. The application of such data to driving rests on the assumption that the pattern of death, morbidity and immediate incapacity are all linked, and hence the stratification of risk from death or hospital admission also applies to sudden short-term incapacity. While there may be some justification for this assumption for atheromatous disease, it is inapplicable to the assessment of potentially disabling but otherwise benign arrhythmias.

Evidence – recurrence of cardiac events[6]

- Recurrence rates can be used as a proxy to stratify risk because of their association with sudden incapacitation. However, measures of recurrence such as death or hospital admission have only limited predictive value for driving.

- Extrapolations to stratify driving risk can be made from large population studies. Most of these data are old and the frequency of recurrence has fallen as a result of better therapy. More recent studies are of highly selected patient groups participating in studies on intervention. It is not possible to extrapolate in a valid way from their recurrence rates to the generality of drivers.

- The older studies identified predictors of recurrence such as poor exercise ECG performance, reduced ventricular ejection fraction, presence of type 2 diabetes and a failure to reduce risk factors.

- A cardiac event makes impairment from vascular disease elsewhere, eg intermittent claudication, stroke or TIA, more likely because the pathological processes are the same. Similarly, ischaemic disease elsewhere increases the probability of a cardiac event.

After most discrete events, the risk of a further episode or of complications is highest in the first hours or days and then progressively reduces, although it rarely falls to the level in those without a prior cardiac event. The pattern of reducing risk is common to several forms of acute coronary syndrome, including myocardial infarction. Data from population studies show that good performance on certain investigations, notably the Bruce protocol exercise ECG, are valid predictors of prognosis, as are scans where pharmacological stress is used to investigate ventricular function. Imaging of structure alone, as in angiography to look for vessel narrowing or occlusion, is less reliable.[7] The use of functional tests even when the presenting disease affects blood vessels distant from the heart, as in stroke or intermittent claudication, has a valid basis because the disease processes of atherosclerotic arterial disease are equally likely to be present in the heart and cause subsequent immediate incapacity from damage there.

Angina

The pain from angina while driving is likely to cause impairment. As it is a consequence of the same disease processes that cause acute cardiac events and strokes, angina is an indicator of an increased risk of future incapacitation.

Arrhythmias

The risks from disorders of cardiac rhythm have rather different features, although many in older people are attributable to ischaemic disease.[8] Some of the ventricular arrhythmias can be life-threatening, and hence may be a cause of death at the wheel, but the more common atrial arrhythmias are either noticed because of slowing or irregularity of the pulse or because of transient faintness or collapse from reduction in cardiac output. Such symptoms have been identified as being relatively common in one study of patients with atrial arrhythmias referred for catheter ablation.[9] As most arrhythmias are recurrent and associated with effects of predictable severity in an individual, past patterns can be used to predict future disabling episodes. The effectiveness of treatment, whether medical or surgical, is assessed in the same way, except that there is a short-term increase in risk immediately after a procedure, such as catheter ablation, pacemaker implant, or a change in treatment.

Arrhythmias and driving risk[10]

Risk is determined by:

- frequency of arrhythmia
- time course of arrhythmia and any provoking factors
- presence of warning symptoms
- likelihood of arrhythmia resulting in loss of consciousness
- likelihood of impaired cognition or distracting symptoms
- risk of event leading to crash.

Evidence – arrhythmias and driving[11]

- Data linking arrhythmias to crashes or citations are not available.
- Impairing symptoms while driving in individuals with recurrent arrhythmias have been reported.
- The risk of recurrence of ventricular arrhythmia is highest in the first few months after the initial episode and then declines (from approximately 4% in the first month to approximately 0.6% per month between 8 and 12 months).
- Implantable cardioverters/defibrillator devices (ICDs) treat ventricular arrhythmias effectively but can be acutely disabling because of the shock delivered while doing so. The probability of discharge depends on the recurrence rate for the arrhythmia, and

a long period without discharge is the best predictor of a low probability of future incapacitation from the device.

- The prevalence of atrial fibrillation/flutter is strongly related to age (>10% over the age of 80). Episodic impairment is usually from fatigue or dizziness. The increased risk of stroke (an approximately five-fold increase) makes this an additional cause of sudden impairment while driving.
- Severe forms of heart block impair safe driving because of syncopal symptoms from reduced cardiac output. Pacemakers are very reliable, with failure rare if the unit is regularly checked.

The disturbing and potentially incapacitating effects of discharge from an implanted defibrillator mean that the probability of discharge while driving is one of the determinants of incapacity. As such machines log discharges, the pattern of recorded discharge can be used to estimate future risks of incapacity. This is relevant to all types of defibrillator – when used for antitachycardia pacing or for shock therapy to convert ventricular arrhythmias.

Hypertension

The relevant risks from hypertension mainly relate to the increased frequency of cardiac events and strokes, if the condition is inadequately treated. Any disabling symptoms from antihypertensive medication may also increase risks. Hypertension has been found to be associated with cognitive impairment and is a major risk factor for vascular dementia.[12]

Aneurysms, aortic dissection and Marfan's syndrome

The risks from these conditions are of rupture, further extension and bleeding. Marfan's syndrome is a risk factor for the development of aneurysms, as well as for ocular pathology. The risk of rupture and sudden bleeding from descending aortic aneurysms is related to their diameter and this may be used as a means of stratifying risk.

Other cardiovascular disorders

For most other cardiovascular disorders, absence of symptoms equates with a low level of risk while driving. These disorders include:

- the cardiomyopathies (unless there is a family history of sudden premature death, or other indicators of an excess risk of sudden incapacity, such as arrhythmias or left ventricular hypertrophy)
- heart and heart/lung transplants (with good exercise capacity)
- heart valve disease (unless with a history of embolism)
- heart failure (with good exercise capacity and left ventricular ejection fraction in excess of 0.4)
- congenital heart disease that is not severe or has been effectively treated.

Clinical assessment and advice

There are marked differences in the fitness criteria applied to Group 1 and Group 2 drivers.[13] This is to an extent derived from an analogy with the criteria used for seizure risk and driving. Thus few cardiovascular conditions are thought to have a risk of such sudden incapacity that it would have the potential to cause immediate incapacitation of more than 20% per annum – the Group 1 criterion for seizures. Many more are considered likely to have risks of more than 2% per annum – the seizure level used as the Group 2 threshold.

Criteria for Group 2 have moved over the past two decades from a highly restrictive approach for all cardiovascular conditions to one where the risk is, where possible, stratified and those in the lower risk groups are permitted to continue driving (Figure 19.1).[14] Predictive assessment using successful completion of the Bruce protocol exercise ECG test as the criterion for a low risk of a recurrence of a cardiac event plays a major part and this may be supplemented by other investigations.[15] However, some conditions remain a bar to driving. For Group 2 drivers all cardiovascular conditions other than hypertension (<180/100 mmHg) should be notified to the DVLA.

Cardiovascular disease is one of the most common reasons for loss of a Group 2 licence. Early advice on controlling risk factors in truck and bus drivers will, if followed, reduce the chances of an early termination of their career.

For Group 1 drivers there are fewer restrictions, mainly based on the time since the last event or the frequency of disabling incidents.

Advice to car drivers should be based on an assessment of:

- *The existence or risk of disabling symptoms while driving*:
  —arrhythmia: distraction or faintness
  —angina: pain (driving must cease if the driver experiences symptoms when at rest or while driving)
  —implanted defibrillator: discharge and pain/muscle contractions.
  A lack of disabling symptoms in the past from the condition is often a useful indicator of a low probability of sudden disability in the future,
- *The presence of impairment without clear symptoms*: cognitive impairment with heart failure, severe hypertension or after major cardiac surgery. Fatigue, particularly if associated with demanding tasks.
- *The risk of sudden incapacity from myocardial infarction or other cardiac event*. This will be increased if there are one or more of the following:
  —prior cardiac event
  —other indications of severe atheromatous disease – angina, stroke or TIA, intermittent claudication
  —surgery for arterial disease – angioplasty, stenting, coronary artery bypass graft
  —tests of cardiac function and reserve, such as the Bruce protocol exercise test, stress myocardial perfusion scanning or

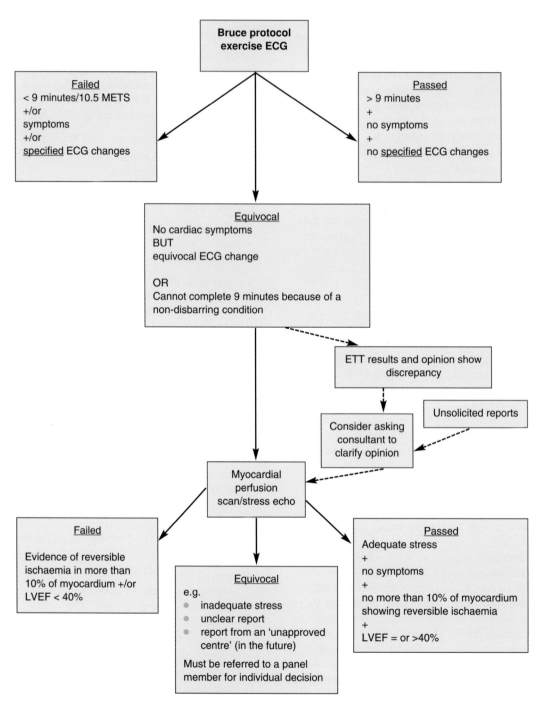

Figure 19.1
Decision tree used by DVLA to assess return to driving after a cardiac event in a Group 2 driver.

stress echocardiography, which show limited cardiac function or reserve. (Imaging of structures, eg with angiography, is a less valid predictor of risk than assessing function)

—continuing presence of cardiac risk factors, such as smoking, high blood pressure, poor lipid profile, diabetes and obesity.

- *The use of any medication*, eg for the treatment of hypertension or arrhythmias, that has the potential to cause disabling symptoms. Experience in use should be used as a guide once treatment has been stabilized.

- Most other cardiovascular conditions, apart from abdominal aortic aneurysms of more than 5.5 cm with their attendant risk of bleeding, provided they are asymptomatic, need not be considered as risks for car drivers.

For Group 1 (car etc.) drivers, notification to the DVLA is only currently required for insertion of a left ventricular assist device, arrhythmia with distracting or disabling symptoms, pacemaker and defibrillator implantation, complete heart block and aortic aneurysm. The overriding legal requirement is a prohibition on driving if 'liable to sudden disabling attacks of dizziness or faintness'.

For other conditions, certain periods of driving cessation after an event or procedure are specified.[16] Notification to the DVLA is not required for Group 1 drivers unless there is another disqualifying condition:

- angioplasty – at least one week
- coronary artery bypass graft (CABG) – at least four weeks
- acute coronary syndromes including myocardial infarction: myocardial infarction – at least four weeks; angioplasty for non-ST elevation myocardial infarction – cease for one week
- arrhythmia – if it is likely to cause incapacity, cease driving for four weeks after the cause has been identified and controlled

- pacemaker implant – at least one week
- successful catheter ablation – at least one week
- prophylactic ICD implant (not one inserted for symptomatic arrhythmia) – one month, but see other DVLA criteria.[16]

If DVLA notification is required, the driver must be informed of their duty to notify and subsequently be asked to confirm when they have done so. In other cases where times are specified for return to driving, these times should form the basis for advice. Over and above these licensing requirements, recommendations to an individual should be based on a clinical assessment of their present state and the probability of any acutely disabling event in the future.

References

1. Dobbs BM. *Medical Conditions and Driving: A Review of the Literature 1960–2000*. DOT HS 809 690. Washington, DC: National Highway Transportation Safety Administration, 2005: 23. www.nhtsa.dot.gov/people/injury/research/MedicalConditions_Driving.pdf

2. Charlton J, et al. *Influence of Chronic Illness on Crash Involvement of Motor Vehicle Drivers*. Report No. 213. Accident Research Centre, Monash University, 2004: 46–89. www.monash.edu.au/muarc/reports/muarc213.pdf

3. *Safe Mobility for Older Drivers. IA1(g) Cardiac and Cardiopulmonary Disorders*. Washington, DC: National Highway Transportation Safety Administration, 2000: 14–17. www.nhtsa.dot.gov/people/injury/olddrive/safe/safe-toc.htm

4. Petch MC. Driving and heart disease: task force report. *Eur Heart J* 1988; **19**: 1165–1177.

5. Dobbs BM. *Medical Conditions and Driving: A Review of the Literature 1960–2000*. DOT HS 809 690. Washington, DC: National Highway Transportation Safety Administration, 2005: 22–24. www.nhtsa.dot.gov/people/injury/research/MedicalConditions_Driving.pdf

6. Joy M, ed. Second European workshop in aviation cardiology. *Eur Heart J* 1999; **1** (Suppl. D).

7. *Expert Consensus Workshop: Driving Safety and Cardiac Ischaemia*. Road Safety Research Report No. 67. London: Department for Transport, 2006. www.dft.gov.uk/stellent/groups/dft_rdsafety/documents/divisionhomepage/030264.hcsp

8. Binns H, Camm J. Driving and arrhythmias (editorial). *BMJ* 2002; **342**: 927–928.

9. Walfridsson U, Walfridsson H. The impact of supraventricular tachycardias on driving ability in patients referred for radiofrequency catheter ablation. *Pacing Clin Electrophysiol* 2005: **28**: 191–195.

10. Dobbs BM. *Medical Conditions and Driving: A Review of the Literature 1960–2000*. DOT HS 809 690. Washington, DC: National Highway Transportation Safety Administration, 2005: 25. www.nhtsa.dot.gov/people/injury/research/ MedicalConditions_Driving.pdf

11. ibid: 26–28.

12. ibid: 31–32.

13. *British Heart Foundation Factfile 07/2000. Driving and the Heart: 1 – Ordinary Driving Licences. Factfile 08/2000. Driving and the Heart: 2 – Vocational Driving Licences.* www.bhf.org.uk

14. Petch MC. Fitness to drive and heart disease. *Proc R Coll Physicians Edin* 1999; **29**: 34–42.

15. Hill J, Timmis A. Exercise tolerance testing. *BMJ* 2002; **342**: 1084–1087.

16. Cardiovascular conditions. *At A Glance Guide*. Swansea: DVLA. www.dvla.gov.uk/at_a_glance/ch2_cardiovascular.htm

20. Diabetes

Impairment and risk
Clinical assessment and advice

Impairment and risk

The most important safety-critical impairment is *hypoglycaemia* (hypo), almost always as a complication of insulin treatment, but occasionally from oral antidiabetic medications, especially sulphonylureas.

Cognitive impairment from hypoglycaemia (prior to incapacitation)

- slower reaction time
- slowed speed of performance of complex tasks
- difficulty in rapid decision-taking
- difficulty with sustained attention
- difficulty with the analysis of complex visual stimuli
- impaired hand–eye coordination
- impaired contrast sensitivity
- mood changes, including tenseness, tiredness, increased anger and irritability
- mental confusion

Other relevant impairments are:

- *Visual loss from cataracts or retinopathy.* The current state of vision should always be considered and this may determine the frequency of follow-up (see p. 71).

- *Loss of sensation and proprioception in the feet from sensory neuropathy* (see p. 98) which may limit the effectiveness of car control, especially if there is coexisting motor weakness or if proprioception and touch sensation prevent effective and timely use of foot pedals. Associated ulceration, gangrene or amputation may prevent driving or require modification to vehicle controls (see p. 49).

- *The excess risk of cardiovascular disease* (see p. 136) *and stroke* (see p. 93).

Other complications such as hyperglycaemia and renal disease do not lead to sudden incapacitation, but hyperglycaemia can cause some cognitive impairment and mood changes.

Evidence – hypoglycaemia and other aspects of diabetes [1–3]

- Impairment from hypoglycaemia (hypo) is complex.

- There is good evidence that mild hypoglycaemia (3–4 mmol/l) induces cognitive impairment. This may cause slowing of response, poor judgement of risk or behavioural changes with increased aggression and risk-taking. It can also blunt awareness of and responses to the warning signs of low blood glucose. [4]

- More severe reductions in blood glucose can lead to frank incapacity and loss of consciousness.

- Perception of early symptoms of a hypo may diminish over time. Early identification of a hypo greatly reduces the risk of consequential crash damage, as either oral carbohydrates can be taken to remedy the hypo or driving ceased. The time course from first awareness to incapacity is variable over a period of seconds to minutes. [5,6]

- Recovery time following a remedy is, in subjective terms, rapid, but there is measurable cognitive impairment for a period of up to 60 minutes or more, suggesting that return to driving should not be immediate. [7]

- Among those at risk of hypoglycaemia the probability of an episode and its severity vary widely. There is currently little valid information that can be used to stratify and predict risk based on age, the duration and severity of the diabetes or the dose or regimen of insulin.

- Hypoglycaemia while driving is not uncommon. As many as 32% of insulin users reported that they had experienced hypoglycaemia while driving, 13% in the previous year. Eighty-nine per cent stated that they would stop driving immediately to treat a hypo.[8]

- There is evidence that, at least for the first few years on insulin, those who have type 2 diabetes are at lower risk than those with type 1 diabetes.

- An individual who has a pattern of repeated reductions in blood glucose on blood glucose monitoring, but is without symptoms, is more likely to have a severe hypoglycaemic episode than someone who has a stable blood glucose level.

- Personal behavioural aspects pose one of the largest problems in determining individual risk. Someone who is careful about maintaining the control of their diabetes, manages it assiduously and does not let the pressures of life or work override its management is likely to be able to maintain far more predictable blood glucose control than someone with irregular eating, activity and monitoring habits.

- There are population-based studies indicating that drivers with diabetes as a group do not have an excess risk of vehicle crashes; these studies do not include fatal accidents.

- However, the DVLA receives a regular flow of police reports of episodes of hypoglycaemia that lead to serious and fatal accidents.

- Clinical assessment of fitness to drive and the advice given depend on careful assessment of the individual.

The risks relevant to driving from other effects of diabetes are not so well established.

Clinical assessment and advice

At initial diagnosis a decision will be taken on the therapy that is required. It is usually the therapy rather than the disease that will determine driving risks. Drivers of Group 2 vehicles must notify the DVLA on diagnosis, while Group 1 drivers need to notify the DVLA if they are on oral antidiabetic medication or insulin.

- Treatment by diet alone has no immediate implications for driving. The loss of a licence that may arise if insulin therapy is required, especially in a vocational driver, may be used as an argument to motivate good compliance with the dietary regimen. Diabetes-related eye conditions, such as cataract and the early stages of retinopathy, may be present, and vision testing to ensure there is no impairment to driving from this cause should be undertaken and repeated regularly.

- The same is usually true if oral antidiabetic medication gives adequate control, although the sulphonylureas may occasionally cause symptomatic hypos. Visual problems become a bigger risk in the long term. It will also be important to advise that, should a change to insulin be indicated, there is likely to be a period when car driving is restricted and driving large vehicles will be permanently prohibited.

- The start of insulin treatment will signal the need both to make a rigorous assessment of fitness to drive and to give specific advice to the patient. Advice should include the statutory requirement placed on drivers to notify the DVLA, which will make further enquiries of the individual and frequently their medical advisers. Particularly in vocational drivers, conflict may arise between giving a treatment regimen that includes insulin and which is best for the individual's long-term health, and maintaining oral treatment to enable them to continue in their current employment. A number of employers who consider that drivers with diabetes, even in small vehicles, pose an excess risk to others may also have internal policies about fitness to drive when on insulin (see Chapter 7).

- Special considerations apply where insulin is used temporarily in certain circumstances, such as after a myocardial infarction and during pregnancy. The implications for driving of new modes of delivery of insulin, such as infusion pumps, preparations for inhalation, etc, have yet to be evaluated and they should be considered in the same way as the injection route.

Patients should be advised to stop driving until insulin doses and glycaemic control have been stabilized. Once stabilization is achieved, car drivers should be advised that they may restart driving subject to the DVLA's response. Drivers of large vehicles who are newly placed on insulin will require vocational guidance, as their Group 2 licence will no longer be valid. Certain drivers of medium-sized commercial vehicles (3.5–7.5 tonnes) may be eligible to continue to hold a licence, but this will depend on an individual assessment after a period of proven good control; hence time away from work can be anticipated.

Labelling of insulin

Your ability to concentrate or react may be reduced if you have hypoglycaemia. Please keep this possible problem in mind in all situations where you might put yourself and others at risk (eg driving a car or operating machinery). You should contact your doctor about the advisability of driving if you have:

- frequent episodes of hypoglycaemia
- reduced or absent warning signs of hypoglycaemia.

Fitness criteria are based on current evidence, which does not allow risk levels for hypoglycaemia to be reliably stratified, based on either age, stage of disease or history of glycaemic control. As and when the risk levels

for hypoglycaemia can be stratified, it may be possible to redefine criteria based on better predictors of individual risk.[9]

- An individual's record of blood glucose measurements, reported frequency of hypos and awareness of falling blood glucose levels are all important factors in assessing fitness. This normally requires the opinion of a diabetologist and may be the approach required by the DVLA in some cases.
- Where the clinician recognizes that glycaemic control is poor and the risk of a hypo is increased, either from blood glucose monitoring results or from impaired awareness of the early signs of hypoglycaemia, the driver should be advised to notify the licensing authority and not to drive until this problem is resolved.
- Similarly, when control may be put at risk by a change in dose or in the insulin formulation prescribed, the need for a temporary halt to driving should be considered.
- There is a conflict between the evidence that strict control of blood glucose reduces the frequency of complications from diabetes but increases the frequency of hypos. This conflict has to be recognized and handled as part of the contract between clinician and patient.
- Careful consideration of timing of food and insulin use may enable drivers using insulin to reduce the risk of hypos at times when driving takes place.
- Driving has its own metabolic demands for glucose, and measurement of blood glucose before driving is recommended. This has been an important legal issue in a number of recent court cases where major accidents have been attributed to hypoglycaemia.[8] Self-recording meters have important advantages in this situation. The use of all types of meters can be monitored from information on the frequency of prescriptions for consumables, and available information suggests they are often underused.

Insulin-using drivers should be given clear advice not just on monitoring but also on:

- the importance of special care if insulin, sleep or meal schedules have been disrupted prior to the drive
- recognition of the increased risk if an individual has taken unusual exercise prior to driving: sport, hard walking or gardening, heavy DIY or manual handling
- the importance of building meal breaks into the schedule for a journey and at the appropriate times
- the need to have carbohydrates in the car for emergency use or in case of delay
- the importance of carrying remedies, either sugar sources or glucagon, for treating hypos
- above all, the requirement to cease driving, remove car keys and move out of the driver's seat in the event of early signs of a hypo or any personal suspicions of impairment to safe driving. Driving should not be re-started until 45 minutes after the blood glucose has risen above 4.0 mmol/l. It may be helpful for regular passengers to be aware of this and to encourage a climate in which they can comment and secure a response from the driver (as with the co-pilot in a plane)
- the benefits of carrying a card or token indicating their condition in the event of unconsciousness.

And on two legal aspects:

- Drivers must be aware that *insulin is just another impairing drug in the eyes of the law (Road Traffic Act 1988)* and that in the event of police involvement they can be prosecuted for driving under its influence.
- Drivers must also be aware that it is their *legal responsibility (Road Traffic Act 1988) to notify the DVLA.* Failure to do so may invalidate their insurance. If they have a contract of employment that requires either a valid licence to be held or unfitness to be declared, they will also be in breach of this.

Thus, in the case of the use of insulin to control diabetes, more than for most other conditions the responsibility for detailed day-to-day management to minimize the risks of a crash while driving rests almost entirely with the driver.

Given observance of these precautions, the vast majority of insulin-using car drivers can continue to drive safely. Regular monitoring is, however, required. In the short term, this is for the driver; in the medium term, it involves both the driver and their clinician – who always needs to consider driving as a part of a consultation; and in the long term, the DVLA by means of decisions about licensing. Diabetes charities provide excellent information to members on safe driving, employment and many other matters (www.diabetes.org.uk).

References

1. Charlton J, *et al. Influence of Chronic Illness on Crash Involvement of Motor Vehicle Drivers.* Report No. 213. Accident Research Centre, Monash University, 2004: 148–154. www.monash.edu.au/muarc/reports/muarc213.pdf

2. Dobbs BM. *Medical Conditions and Driving: A Review of the Literature 1960–2000.* DOT HS 809 690. Washington, DC: National Highway Transportation Safety Administration, 2005: 80–88. www.nhtsa.dot.gov/people/injury/research/MedicalConditions_Driving.pdf

3. *Safe Mobility for Older Drivers. IA1(c) Diabetes.* Washington, DC: National Highways Transportation Safety Administration, 2000: 7–10. www.nhtsa.dot.gov/people/injury/olddrive/safe/safe-toc.htm

4. Deary IJ. Symptoms of hypoglycaemia and effects on mental performance and emotions. In: Frier B, Fisher BM, eds. *Hypoglycaemia and Clinical Diabetes.* Chichester: John Wiley, 1991: 29–54.

5. Frier B, Fisher BM. Impaired hypoglycaemia awareness. In: Frier B, Fisher BM, eds. *Hypoglycaemia and Clinical Diabetes.* Chichester: John Wiley, 1991: 111–146.

6. MacLeod K. Hypoglycaemia unawareness: causes, consequences and treatment. *J R Coll Phys Lond* 2000; **34**: 245–250

7. Evans ML, Pernet A, Lomas J, *et al.* Delay in onset of awareness of acute hypoglycaemia and of restoration of cognitive performance during recovery. *Diabetes Care* 2000; **23**: 893–897.

8. Graveling A, Warren R, Frier B. Hypoglycaemia and driving in people with insulin treated diabetes: adherence to recommendations for avoidance. *Diabetic Med* 2003; **21**: 1014–1019.

9. Heller S, *et al. Stratifying Hypoglycaemia Risk in Insulin Treated Diabetes*. Road Safety Research Report 61. London: Department for Transport, 2006. www.dft.gov.uk/stellent/groups/dft_rdsafety/documents/ divisionhomepage/030264.hcsp

21. Sleep disorders

Impairment and risk
Clinical assessment and advice

Impairment and risk

Sleep and accidents

Loss of consciousness through falling asleep while driving is an important cause of crashes.

- Two medical conditions, narcolepsy and obstructive sleep apnoea (OSA), commonly result in excessive daytime sleepiness and contribute to such accidents. Drivers with these conditions have an excess risk of crashes.

- Other medical causes for recurrent sleep disturbance, such as 'restless legs syndrome,' pain or chronic cough, or insomnia associated with mental ill-health can all, if severe enough, lead to excessive daytime sleepiness.

- However, the majority of sleep-related crashes are not in people with predisposing conditions but in drivers, largely young males, who are sleep deprived and who fall asleep while driving at night.

- In older drivers, as well as nocturnal sleepiness, there can be a marked period of excessive drowsiness in the afternoon, resulting in a smaller but observable excess of crashes.

This has implications for road safety policy in that to reduce accidents the emphasis is rightly on 'don't drive sleepy' and 'if you are tired take a break.' This is also rational in that most of those with sleep disorders experience similar warnings to others who are in danger of falling asleep, although they may be habituated to them from continued tiredness, or these warning signals may only be present for a short period before unconsciousness occurs.

As tiredness increases, driving performance deteriorates, particular features of which are:

- a tendency to be late in correcting car direction, with large infrequent steering movements

- a degree of cognitive impairment which results in the warning symptoms of impending sleep being ignored

- the level of external stimulation is important. Sleep-related crashes (which can be identified by the vehicle slowly veering from its course, without correction and without any braking applied until it crashes) are most frequent on tedious roads with little stimulation from traffic conditions

- drivers do not reliably remember short periods of sleep and readily forget even the sensation of sleepiness after the stimulation and distress of a crash

- taking a break, a brief doze and caffeine all help to reduce the impairment arising from one night's sleep deprivation, which is equivalent to that from the maximum acceptable level of blood alcohol.[1]

Evidence – sleepiness and road safety

- It is estimated that around 300 people a year are killed because a driver has fallen asleep at the wheel. Around 40% of sleep-related crashes involve commercial vehicles. This type of accident is most frequent on motorways and similar roads. Men under 30 years of age have the highest risk of sleep-related crashes.[2]

- Estimates of the proportion of accidents attributable to sleep vary widely: USA 1–3%, France 10%, Australia 30%, UK police reports 16–20%, driver reports 9–10%.

- The proportion of accidents related to specific sleep disorders is not known, but 33% of these individuals had had traffic accidents in the past five years, while

19–27% admitted to having fallen asleep at the wheel. One study indicates an accident rate of 13 per million kilometres for those with a sleep disorder, compared to 0.8 for a control group.[3]

Obstructive sleep apnoea (OSA)

This is the most common sleep disorder. Sleep becomes fragmented because of intermittent obstruction of the airway in the neck during sleep, leading to hypoxia and awakening to clear the airway. This may happen many times an hour during sleep. As a consequence there is marked daytime sleepiness and it is this which is a risk while driving.

OSA is most common in middle-aged males; it is associated with obesity and large neck size. Given the at-risk population, truck and coach drivers are not uncommonly affected, and in the event of a crash may cause considerable consequential damage and injury. There are a number of treatments for OSA aimed at maintaining an open airway. The most common is the use of a continuous positive airways pressure (CPAP) machine at night. Newer machines log the timing of use as an aid to compliance assessment. These improve the quality of sleep and thus reduce daytime sleepiness. Splints to advance the mandible and other methods of treatment are also sometimes used. Weight loss and abstention from alcohol may also reduce the severity of the condition.

Evidence – obstructive sleep apnoea [4]

- Cognitive deficits are found in those with sleep apnoea. It is not clear whether these are fatigue-related or whether they are a specific effect of recurring hypoxia.
- A number of studies have shown an increased rate both of sleep-related and of total crashes. Most studies have flaws in their design, in particular a lack of diagnostic criteria and absence of correction for distance driven.
- Driving simulator studies show reduced performance.

- Studies investigating the relationship between the severity of the condition and crashes or simulator performance have not given consistent results.
- Opinion is divided on whether there is the same warning pattern of sleepiness prior to loss of consciousness as in the general population.
- Treatment with CPAP has been shown to reduce both crashes and errors made during simulated driving.
- There are no studies of the effect of other forms of treatment on driving.
- Because of the age group and lifestyle characteristics of the highest risk group (<2% of the general population but 8% of middle-aged men) for sleep apnoea, co-morbidity is common.

Narcolepsy

This is a rare genetically linked condition, with profound sleepiness during the day despite sleeping at night. Sudden 'sleep attacks' may occur. It is usually associated with cataplexy – sudden weakness and collapse, sometimes in association with an emotion such as laughter in response to an external event. Stimulants used in treatment can reduce the severity of daytime symptoms. There is an obvious risk in driving when liable to sudden sleep or weakness, but there are no specific studies on narcolepsy and crashes or driving performance.

Clinical assessment and advice

Because of the well-established excess crash risk in those with sleep disorders, a high index of suspicion is needed, especially in those who drive large vehicles for long distances and have inflexible driving schedules.[5] The medical examination for holders of Group 2 licences now includes specific questions about sleep patterns and daytime sleepiness. It is good practice to ask similar questions in others at high risk, such as overweight middle-aged males, as a routine. Some operators of bus and truck fleets, and organizations with large numbers of on-the-road staff, have training and awareness programmes about tiredness, sleep disorders and driving to help their drivers recognize these problems. Vehicle damage and accidents may also be investigated with this in mind.

Recognition of sleep disorders, in particular OSA, is not always straightforward. Fatigue or other somatic symptoms may be reported, but the individual may be unaware of just how disrupted their nocturnal sleep is. Partners or others who have witnessed them sleeping are often able to confirm the characteristic recurrent pattern of apnoea and then gasping. Symptoms may be attributed to ageing and may not be fully revealed if the individual is worried about their employment prospects.

Information to be elicited in assessing whether there may be a sleep-related risk while driving includes:

- perceived quality of night-time sleep and whether the individual feels refreshed in the morning
- any comments from others about the individual snoring, struggling and gasping during the night
- prolonged periods of kicking (lower legs) or creeping/crawling sensations in legs (usually thighs) around sleep onset and during sleep
- tendency to fall asleep when sitting quietly
- episodes of sleepiness while concentration is needed, eg driving
- time taken to fall asleep.

The Epworth sleepiness scale may be used for assessing sleep disorders, and it may be coupled with supplementary questions to determine risk factors for sleep apnoea and other disorders (see p. 162). All forms of questioning depend on subjective perceptions and on a willingness to admit to a problem. Information on crashes or near misses can supplement self-perceptions, but further investigations may be needed.

Investigation may be undertaken, including overnight sleep studies by a sleep specialist. Questionnaires and outpatient testing may also provide useful diagnostic information. A successful trial of CPAP therapy may also help confirm the presence of OSA.

All drivers with diagnosed sleep disorders should inform the DVLA. If there are strong suspicions of a sleep disorder, especially in a Group 2 driver or in someone who has to drive for long hours as a part of their work, then cessation of driving and notification of the DVLA need to be recommended. Referral to a sleep clinic should also be arranged, as it is likely that its specialist recommendations will be needed before driving is resumed.

Resumption of driving in the case of OSA may well be dependent on continued use of CPAP, preferably a machine that is able to log use, so that, in the event of an accident, compliance with the requirement to use CPAP can be confirmed. The reduction in risk may be sufficient for the individual to resume driving all classes of vehicle. In some people with narcolepsy, the regular use of stimulant medications or other psychoactive drugs can reduce the incidence of sudden daytime sleepiness. This reduction in risk may enable resumption of driving a car, but not a larger vehicle. The disabling effects of any associated cataplexy and the effectiveness of its treatment also have to be taken into account.

Drivers should be made aware that there have been successful prosecutions of those who knew that they had subjective symptoms of a sleep disorder or who had not complied with recommendations for investigation and treatment. These prosecutions have been for careless and dangerous driving because the defendants were not fit to drive on account of their recurrent tendency to disabling daytime sleepiness.

References

1. Williamson AM, Feyer A-M. Moderate sleep deprivation produces impairments in cognitive and motor performance equivalent to legally prescribed levels of alcohol intoxication. *Occup Environ Med* 2000; **57**: 649–655.

2 Road Safety Reports 22 and 52. www.dft.gov.uk/stellent/groups/dft_rdsafety/documents/ divisionhomepage/ 030261.hcsp

3. Horstmann S, Hess CW, Bassetti C, *et al*. Sleepiness-related accidents in sleep apnoea patients. *Sleep* 2000; **23**: 383–389.

4. Charlton J, et al. *Influence of Chronic Illness on Crash Involvement of Motor Vehicle Drivers*. Report No. 213. Accident Research Centre, Monash University, 2004: 330–343. www.monash.edu.au/muarc/reports/muarc213.pdf

5. Carter T, Major H, Wetherall G, Nicholson A. Excessive daytime sleepiness and driving: regulations for road safety. *Clin Med* 2004; **4**: 454–456.

Appendix 1: Tools for assessment of fitness to drive

Older drivers (AMA)
Dementia (CDR, Ottawa, Hartford)
Retiring from driving
Sleep questionnaires
Alcohol questionnaire

Older drivers (AMA)

Assessment of capacity for car driving (older driver): The American Medical Association (AMA) and the US National Highway Transportation Safety Agency

These bodies have recently proposed a set of assessments that they consider are a good starting point for a health professional who is advising the older driver on whether they can continue to drive or whether they should seek a more specialized appraisal of their capability.

The assessment uses techniques that are readily performed in a surgery or outpatient setting. Each has some evidence of validity in distinguishing between drivers at high and at low risk of crashes or poor simulator performance. The validity of the battery as a whole has not been proven. All tests can be explained to the patient as being relevant to the driving task, and vision, cognition and motor performance are all assessed.

This assessment is included in an online publication, *Assessing and Counseling Older Drivers*, which has many parallels to this book, but which is written for a federal country where statutory criteria for fitness to drive vary considerably between states.[1] It is also set in a style of medical practice where regular physician check-ups are normal and hence where such testing can readily be seen as an extension of this routine. Despite these differences from Britain in driver regulation and healthcare practice, the approach is a useful one for helping to resolve questions or concerns about fitness to drive addressed to the health professional.

Assessment of driving-related skills (ADReS)

The driver needs to be engaged in the process of assessment. Answering questions about driving prior to the health professional's assessment is a useful start (see Am I a safe driver, p. 155). The terminology has been modified to British usage. Answers should be seen as a prompt to further enquiry rather than as a definitive statement, and need to be interpreted in the light of any parallel observations about insight and recall.

The assessment forms part of a wider process for deciding if the patient is at risk from medically impaired driving (Figure A1.1). It includes:

- visual acuity (Snellen) and fields (confrontation)
- cognition by executive task (trail-making test [part B])
- visual–spatial attention (drawing clock)
- endurance (rapid-pace walk)
- range of joint motion (neck, fingers, shoulder/elbow, ankle)
- motor strength (shoulder, hip, wrist, ankle, hand grip).

In conducting the assessment it is important to emphasize that the tests all relate to essential capabilities for driving and that they are a snapshot of how the driver is on the day of testing. They do not in any way predict future performance, although in the main the functions tested are all ones that are either relatively stable or slowly declining in the older driver.

It is suggested that all tests are done with explanation of their relevance to driving but without interpreting the results of each at the time. The results should be recorded to enable future comparisons. The overall results should be discussed with the driver at the end of the assessment.

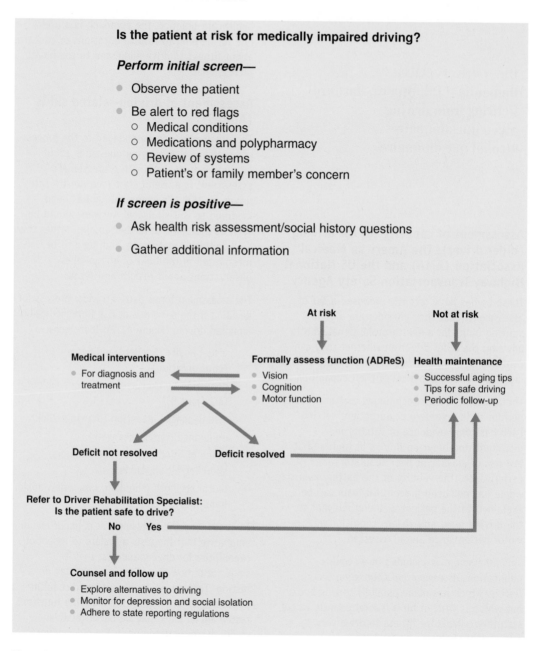

Is the patient at risk for medically impaired driving?

Perform initial screen—

- Observe the patient
- Be alert to red flags
  - Medical conditions
  - Medications and polypharmacy
  - Review of systems
  - Patient's or family member's concern

If screen is positive—

- Ask health risk assessment/social history questions
- Gather additional information

At risk

Not at risk

Medical interventions
- For diagnosis and treatment

Formally assess function (ADReS)
- Vision
- Cognition
- Motor function

Health maintenance
- Successful aging tips
- Tips for safe driving
- Periodic follow-up

Deficit not resolved

Deficit resolved

Refer to Driver Rehabilitation Specialist: Is the patient safe to drive?

No   **Yes**

Counsel and follow up
- Explore alternatives to driving
- Monitor for depression and social isolation
- Adhere to state reporting regulations

Figure A1.1
Older driver assessment flow chart.[1]

Am I a safe driver?

Self-assessment: this will not be disclosed to anyone by your doctor but will help guide their own review of your health and help them to advise you on your driving. Tick the box if the statement applies to you.

- ☐ I get lost while driving.
- ☐ My friends and family members say they are worried about my driving.
- ☐ Other cars seem to appear out of nowhere.
- ☐ I have trouble seeing signs in time to respond to them.
- ☐ Other drivers drive too fast.
- ☐ Other drivers often honk at me.
- ☐ Driving stresses me out.
- ☐ After driving, I feel tired.
- ☐ I have had more 'near misses' lately.
- ☐ Busy intersections bother me.
- ☐ Right-hand turns make me nervous.
- ☐ The glare from oncoming headlights bothers me.
- ☐ My medication makes me dizzy or drowsy.
- ☐ I have trouble turning the steering wheel.
- ☐ I have trouble pushing down on the accelerator or brakes.
- ☐ I have trouble looking over my shoulder when I reverse.
- ☐ I have been stopped by the police for my driving recently.
- ☐ People will no longer accept rides from me.
- ☐ I don't like to drive at night.
- ☐ I have had more trouble parking lately.

If you have ticked any of the boxes, your safety may be at risk when you drive. Talk to your doctor about ways to improve your safety when you drive.

Sensory tests

- Visual acuity (corrected). To best simulate driving, visual requirements use a 6 m Snellen chart. A 3 m chart may, however, be used. The test can be done with both eyes open, as it is the overall acuity that is relevant. It may be worth checking near acuity if the driver complains of problems reading maps or gauges.

1. If less than 6/12 recommend sight test and appropriate correction. If prescribed, glasses should be worn when driving:
  —discuss any visual problems the patient has while driving and recommend ways round them, eg avoiding driving at night or in bad weather
  —ensure there is periodic re-testing and replacement of glasses if indicated.

2. If less than 6/18 in addition to the above, recommend on-road assessment (this reflects US practice. At this level the number plate test will probably be failed and, if this is so, the individual must stop driving and inform the DVLA).

3. If less than 6/24 in addition to the above, cease driving until and unless driving ability can be demonstrated in an on-road assessment (reflects US practice – driving illegal in EU).

- *Visual fields.* The clinical confrontation test (Donders) is not ideal but can serve as an initial screen, with referral to an optometrist if a defect is suspected. Defects in older drivers commonly follow strokes. Each eye should be tested separately at a distance of 3 feet. The examiner's fingers should be correctly counted rather than movement being detected.

Ensure adequate treatment, consider on-road assessment and driver rehabilitation, consider vehicle modifications. Re-test regularly if progressive condition. (This reflects US practice. In the UK, inform the DVLA, which will arrange for an optometrist to undertake perimetry.)

Two other aspects of visual function are often reduced in older drivers:

—contrast sensitivity, especially in low-light conditions, eg unilluminated signs or house numbers at night or low-contrast pedestrians at twilight

—adaptation to changing levels of illumination, eg a long recovery period after facing oncoming headlights. Glare and light scatter from early cataracts may worsen this.

Ask about these problems.

Cognitive tests

A wide range of cognitive skills are needed for driving, including memory, visual processing, division of attention and executive skills. Taken together, the trail-making test (part B) and the clock drawing test are two measures that integrate a number of these functions. Both are simple to score.

- *Trail-making test (part B).* This involves sequentially joining up numbers and letters on a printed sheet.[2] The instructions are, 'Now I will give you a paper and pencil. On the paper are the numbers 1 to 12 and the letters A to L, scattered across the page. Starting with 1 draw a line to A, then to 2 then to B and so on, alternating back and forth between numbers and letters until you finish with the number 12. I will time how fast you can go. Are you ready? Go.' The examiner points out and corrects errors and so this lengthens the test time. The score is the time to complete correctly. *A time to completion of more than 180 seconds signals a need for more detailed intervention (see below).*

- *Clock drawing test.* Give the driver a pencil and a blank sheet of paper and say, 'I would like you to draw the face of a clock, put in all the numbers, and set the time at 10 minutes past 11.' The test is not timed but is scored for eight specific elements:

—all 12 hours are placed in correct numerical order, starting with 12 at the top

—only the numbers 1–12 are included (no duplicates, omissions or foreign marks)

—the number are drawn inside the clock circle

—the numbers are spaced equally or nearly equally from each other

—the numbers are spaced equally or nearly equally from the edge of the circle

—one clock hand points to 2 o'clock

—one clock hand points to 11 o'clock

—there are only two clock hands.

If impaired cognition is detected on either of these tests, further investigation is warranted and should be considered before advising on continuation of driving:

- more detailed tests to assess cognitive impairment
- identification and treatment, where possible, of any medical conditions contributing to impairment. Specialist referral if indicated
- screening for depression
- review of medication regimen to identify any impairing agents
- on-road driving assessment by driving assessor, in particular to look at capacity for sustained attention
- periodic review if condition is progressive.

Motor tests

- *Rapid-pace walking.* A measure of lower limb strength, endurance, range of motion, balance and gross proprioception. A corridor is used with marked start and turning points. The driver is asked to walk a 10 foot path, turn around and walk back to the starting point as quickly as possible. If a stick or frame is normally used, this can be used for the test. It is timed from the first foot being lifted until the finishing line is crossed. *A time of more than 9 seconds indicates a need for further action.*

- *Range of motion.* To assess capabilities with car controls and manoeuvring:
  —neck rotation – 'Look over your shoulder as if you are reversing or parking. Now do the same thing on the other side'
  —finger curl – 'Make fists with both your hands'
  —shoulder and elbow flexion – 'Pretend you are holding the steering wheel.

  Now pretend to make a large right turn, then a large left turn'
  —ankle plantar flexion – 'Pretend you are pressing the accelerator hard; now do the same with the other foot'
  —ankle dorsiflexion – 'Point your toes towards you'

  Record as within or outside normal limits. Outside if range good but hesitation or pain, or if range severely limited.

- *Motor strength.* Tested by manually flexing or extending drivers' limbs and asking them to resist these movements. Bilateral tests of:
  —shoulder adduction, abduction and flexion
  —hip flexion and extension
  —wrist flexion and extension
  —ankle dorsiflexion and plantar flexion
  —hand-grip strength.

  Results graded as 5 – normal, full resistance; 4 – some resistance; 3 – against gravity only; 2 – not against gravity;
  1 – muscle contraction but no movement;
  0 – no contraction no movement.

All these tests of motor function are somewhat subjective but can indicate the need for further advice or action:

- encourage use of vehicle with light controls, steering, brakes, etc and with automatic transmission
- recommend regular regimen of physical activity to maintain fitness to drive, with specific advice or referral if needed
- provide effective, but non-impairing, pain control for musculoskeletal problems
- diagnose and treat any conditions found that potentially interfere with driving
- consider need for on-road expert assessment and advice on modified controls.

If the driver performs well in all sections of the assessment, they can, in the absence of any other problems, be advised that they can continue driving, subject to periodic follow-up.

If they perform poorly but remedial advice or treatment is possible, re-assess once this is in place. Advise on need for self-awareness of any driving problems and modification of driving pattern or cessation if they interfere with safe driving. Expert on-road assessment should be considered if there is uncertainty about safety, if remedial teaching may assist or if vehicle modifications may enable continuation.

If impairments cannot be remedied, counseling about the need to cease driving and the duties of the driver to surrender their licence should be undertaken.

These dialogues are likely to be less effective if there is loss of cognition from a dementing process (see Chapter 10.

Questions about driving[3]

Suggested questions to gain understanding of and build a relationship with the patient as a driver or with concerned relatives are:

- How much do you (or your relative) drive?
- Do you usually have any passengers?
- Do you have any problems when you drive? (Ask specifically about day and night vision, ease of operating steering wheel and foot pedals, confusion and delayed reactions to traffic signs and situations.)
- Do you think you are a safe driver?
- Do you ever get lost while driving?
- Have you been issued with any ticket or warnings in the past two years?
- Have you had any near-misses or crashes in the past two years?

And about wider mobility needs:

- How do you usually get around? Does this work well for you?
- If your car ever broke down, how would you get around?

Encourage discussion of a transport safety net. 'Mobility is very important for your physical and emotional health. If you were ever unable to drive for any reason, I'd want to make certain that you could still keep appointments and pick up medications as well as being able to go shopping for essentials and visit your friends and family.'

Adapted and reproduced with permission from the American Medical Association's *Physician's Guide to Assessing and Counseling Older Drivers*, Washington, DC: National Highways Transportation Safety Administration, 2003

Dementia (CDR, Ottawa, Hartford)

A number of bodies have made recommendations about the role of the health professional in assessing and advising on the early stages of progressive dementia and fitness to drive, and proposed techniques for carrying out this task. To an extent it is simply a subset of the wider process of assessment of the older driver. There are, however, a number of specific aspects that are described below.

The clinical dementia rating (CDR)

This is a tool that has been shown to have some predictive value.[4] Those in category 0.5 show some increase in driving risk but not to a level that is above other higher risk groups of road users, while those in category 2 have an unacceptably high risk.[5]

The driving and dementia toolkit (Ottawa, Canada)

This provides a series of information sheets for patients, families and health professionals.[6] It lists:

1. *Risk factors for driving problems 'SAFEDRIVE:'*

- safety record – recent crashes and near misses
- attention skills – lapses in consciousness or recurrent episodes of confusion
- family record – observations on patient's driving ability
- ethanol – screen for alcohol abuse
- drugs – review medication, checking for sedating or anticholinergic drugs
- reaction time – any neurological or musculoskeletal disorders which may slow reactions
- intellectual impairment – perform Mini Mental State Examination[7,8]
- visual/visual–spatial function – check for visual activity
- executive functions – check ability to plan and sequence activities and self-monitor behaviours.
- If any are positive, seek more detailed assessment.

2. Ten questions to ask the patient:
- Have you noticed any change in your driving skills?
- Do others honk or show signs of irritation?
- Have you lost any confidence in your overall driving ability, leading you to drive less often or only in good weather?
- Have you ever become lost while driving?
- Have you ever forgotten where you were going?
- do you think at present that you are an unsafe driver?
- Have you had any car accidents in the last year?
- Any minor damage (fender-benders) with other cars in car parks (parking lots)?
- Have you received any traffic citations for speeding, going too slow, improper turns, failure to stop, etc.?
- Have others criticized your driving or refused to drive with you?

3. Ten questions to ask the family:
- Do you feel uncomfortable in any way driving with your relative?
- Have you noted any abnormal or unsafe behaviour?
- Has your relative had any recent crashes?
- Has your relative had near-misses that could be attributed to mental or physical decline?
- Has your relative received any tickets or traffic violations?
- Are other drivers forced to drive defensively to accommodate your

relative's errors in judgement?

- Have there been any occasions where your relative has got lost or experienced navigational confusion?

- Does your relative need many cues or directions from passengers?

- Does your relative need a co-pilot* to alert them of potentially hazardous events or conditions?

- Have others commented on your relative's unsafe driving?

  *There is general recognition that dependence on a co-pilot for anything other than advance navigational instructions is not acceptable, as responses to a co-pilot's instructions will be slower and they may create emotional pressures that further interfere with limited perception.

4. What to tell your patients – if you consider that they have early problems but are still fit to drive:
   —drive only on familiar routes
   —drive slowly
   —don't drive at night
   —don't use the radio because it can be distracting
   —avoid busy intersections
   —don't drive with a distracting companion
   —take (relevant older driver training) course
   —avoid motorways
   —avoid rush hour traffic.

5. How to advise a patient that they should cease driving. This aspect relates closely to Canadian and Ontario driver licensing procedures, where the physician has an obligation to report impairing medical conditions and so is not appropriate as advice in Britain.

Reproduced with permission from *The Driving and Dementia Toolkit*. © 2001 Regional Geriatric Assessment Programme of Ottawa – Carleton.

At the Crossroads: a Guide to Alzheimer's Disease, Dementia and Driving.[9]

This publication by a US insurer is a useful source of driver- and family-oriented advice. In particular, it provides cues to some of the difficult questions that a driver who is developing a progressive dementia and their relatives need to address. It includes the following self-assessment form for drivers:

Warning signs for drivers with dementia

1. Have you noticed any of the following warning signs?
2. Is there a change in frequency or severity of these warning signs?
3. Do the circumstances and seriousness of the warning signs warrant continued close monitoring, driving modification or an immediate end to driving?

Warning sign	Date observed	Frequency/notes
Incorrect signalling		
Trouble navigating turns		
Moving into the wrong lane		
Confusion at exits		
Parking inappropriately		
Hitting kerbs		
Failing to notice traffic signs		
Driving at inappropriate speeds		
Delayed responses to unexpected situations		
Not anticipating potentially dangerous situations		
Increased agitation or irritation when driving		
Scrapes or dents on car, garage, etc		
Getting lost in familiar places		
Near misses		
Ticketed moving violations/warnings		
Car accident		
Confusing brake and accelerator pedals		
Stopping in traffic for no apparent reason		
Other signs.........		

Agreement with my family about driving – this pro forma letter is suggested:

To my family

The time may come when I can no longer make the best decisions for the safety of others and myself. Therefore, in order to help my family make necessary decisions, this statement is an expression of my wishes and directions while I am still able to make these decisions.

I have discussed with my family my desire to drive as long as it is safe for me to do so.

When it is not reasonable for me to drive, I desire...[person's name].. to tell me I can no longer drive.

I trust my family will take the necessary steps to prohibit my driving in order to ensure my safety and the safety of others while protecting my dignity.

Signed.................... Date......................

Reproduced with permission from The Hartford Financial Services Group, Inc., *At the Crossroads: A Guide to Alzheimer's Disease, Dementia and Driving*, © 2006 The Hartford, Hartford, CT 06115

Retiring from driving[10]

Advice from a doctor is a common reason for ceasing to drive. It is not always easy advice to give. Its justification needs to be based on the view that the person is a safety risk to themselves and other road users. It should be the advice of last resort only given when remedial measures have been ineffective. It may be better given by a trusted health professional who can advise on alternatives rather than coming as a letter revoking a licence. The latter will usually be as the result of a specific medical condition, though in many older drivers there may not be a single condition leading to a licensing decision but rather increasing frailty, slowing of responses, cognitive impairment and less effective visual and visual–perceptual functioning.

The concept of 'retirement from driving' may be useful. Even raising this may lead to anger or feeling that their trusting relationship with the adviser is being threatened. Often there are severe practical issues, such as the dependence of a spouse or others on their driving for essential mobility. Hence discussion needs to be coupled with a review of alternative transport options and their economics as compared with car ownership. This should include review of the savings from concessionary fares and free travel passes.

These may be introduced by questions such as:

- How do you get around when your car is being serviced?
- Can you then still get everywhere you need to?
- Have you ever thought how you would get around if you couldn't drive?

And by prompting about alternatives, with discussion of any perceived barriers to use:

- walking
- bus or train
- rides from family or friends
- taxis
- dial-a-ride services
- hospital car service

- volunteers from churches, clubs, etc
- use of delivery and on-line shopping
- home visits from service providers
- use of powered aids such as buggies
- house move to more accessible location.

Planning also involves thinking how to combine activities so that a single trip can meet several functions.

Family members often need to participate in the process by:

- understanding and being able to explain the rationale for the recommended retirement from driving
- preferably being present on at least some of the occasions when it is being discussed
- providing resources and help with mobility advice and with actual transport
- helping to sort out reliable options, such as helpful cab drivers/companies and the right relationships with friends and neighbours so that help can continue to be offered and accepted willingly
- recognizing the economic aspects of comparison between the full costs of car ownership and the costs of public transport and taxi use
- make family members aware that they may, if the individual has walking problems, be eligible to use a disabled parking badge when transporting the person.

Reinforcing advice on 'retirement from driving'

- Give the individual the opportunity to ask questions and explain the reasons for your advice.
- Where practicable, engage relatives in the decision.
- Get them to repeat back the reasons why they should not drive.
- Consider giving them a 'prescription' stating 'Do not drive' or sending a confirmatory letter.
- Advise them that they are responsible for

informing the DVLA and follow this up at the next visit.

- Point to the very high costs per mile of car ownership when little use is made of the car, identifying that they will have enough for several taxi journeys a month from the savings of giving up vehicle ownership.

After driving has ceased

This will be a time of adaptation and usually both some practical problems and loss of self-esteem. At any follow-up visits check on this, preferably with a supportive family member present, and ensure that the changes have not precipitated depressive mood changes or unjustified dependency and self-neglect.

Sleep questionnaire

The Epworth Sleepiness Scale is used to determine the level of daytime sleepiness. A score of 10 or more is considered sleepy. A score of 18 or more is very sleepy.

It is designed to be self-completed and may be downloaded from a number of websites.[11]

Alcohol questionnaire

The Gage is a simple questionnaire that asks questions about alcohol use in ways that have been found to be useful predictors of abuse and dependency. It may be downloaded from a number of websites.[12]

References

1. *Physician's Guide to Assessing and Counseling Older Drivers*. Washington, DC: National Highways Transportation Safety Administration, 2003. Chapter 1: 4. www.nhtsa.dot.gov/people/injury/olddrive/ OlderDriversBook/pages/Chapter1.html

2. www.nhtsa.dot.gov/people/injury/olddrive/ OlderDriversBook/pages/Trail-Making.html

3. *Physician's Guide to Assessing and Counseling Older Drivers*. Washington, DC: National Highways Transportation Safety Administration, 2003. Chapter 2: 4. www.nhtsa.dot.gov/people/injury/olddrive/ OlderDriversBook/pages/Chapter2.html

4. Morris JC. The clinical dementia rating (CDR) current version and scoring rules. *Neurology* 1993; **43**: 2412–2414.

5. Brown LB, Ott BR. Driving and dementia: a review of the literature. *J Geriatr Psychiatry Neurol* 2004; **17**: 232–240.

6. *The Driving and Dementia Toolkit*. Regional Geriatric Assessment Programme of Ottawa – Carleton. www.rgapottawa.com/dementia/english/default.asp

7. Mini Mental State Examination. www.rgapottawa.com/dementia/english/forms.asp

8. Folstein M, Folstein SE, McHugh PR. 'Mini-Mental State' a practical method for grading the cognitive state of patients for the clinician. *J Psychiatric Res* 1975; **12**: 189-198

9. *At the Crossroads: A Guide to Alzheimer's Disease, Dementia and Driving*. www.thehartford.com/alzheimers/105013final.pdf

10. *Physician's Guide to Assessing and Counseling Older Drivers*. Washington, DC: National Highway Transportation Safety Administration, Chapter 6: 2–9. www.nhtsa.dot.gov/people/injury/olddrive/ OlderDriversBook/pages/Chapter6.html

11. www.thedoctorwillseeyounow.com/articles/ senior_living/questionnaire_12/epworth.shtml

12. www.thedoctorwillseeyounow.com/articles/ senior_living/questionnaire_12/cage.shtml

Appendix 2: Fitness for other safety-critical tasks

Air pilots
Rail employees
Seafarers
Offshore workers
Divers
Physically demanding public safety work
Control room work

There are a number of other tasks and occupations where impairment due to health can put not only the individual affected but also others at risk. While not the main subject of this book, some of the more important of these activities, the basis for their health-related fitness criteria and the sources of further information are noted as an aid for reference.[1]

There is also a wide range of leisure activities, such as sailing, climbing, flying and diving, where a health problem in one of a team can put others at risk. Most such activities have either formal or informal fitness standards developed by their governing bodies. Those asking for advice should be recommended to obtain these standards and observe them – seeking the support of a health professional as needed.

Air pilots

The Civil Aviation Authority (CAA) is responsible for the arrangements for assessing pilot fitness. Fitness of cabin crew is a matter for airlines, but the CAA has knowledge of company procedures as part of the licensing process for commercial operators. The fitness criteria for commercial and other international pilots (and for air traffic controllers) are compatible in many European Union and certain other European countries and are issued as the Joint Aviation Requirements Flight crew licensing (medical) standards (JAR-FCL 3). These requirements are issued to medical examiners appointed by national authorities such as the CAA. The frequency of medical assessments varies according to age and type of flying, the CAA provides an expert reference service for borderline cases and results are held on a central CAA database, with protected access.

Pilots flying light planes within the UK as well as those involved in other air sports such as ballooning and gliding can choose to have a simpler assessment for a National Private Pilot's Licence in which their general practitioner has to countersign a self-declaration of fitness, using the DVLA Group 1 (for solo flying) and the Group 2 (for flying with passengers) criteria as benchmarks. Air sports governing bodies have medical advisers who decide on any borderline cases and the CAA has oversight of the system.

Rail employees

Industry standards are published by the Rail Safety and Standards Board.[2] These implement a basic legal duty 'to ensure that the fitness and competency of safety-critical workers is assessed and monitored'. Network Rail and the train operating companies make arrangements for medical assessment by occupational health providers, whose medical staff have to meet specified competence requirements. They apply the standards in the light of their clinical findings. The arrangements for determining fitness and competence form an essential part of each operator's safety case. Standards vary with the job, the most stringent applying to drivers and signallers. Train crew have some safety functions; these mainly relate to making a disabled train safe and to evacuating passengers, hence they need a certain level of physical fitness. Line-side workers and others who have to access the tracks need to have the awareness to avoid trains and also have to be capable of working in adverse weather conditions. Line-side workers include a large number engaged by contractors on engineering and maintenance work. A number of these standards, as well as the regulation of rail safety, are likely to change in response to alterations in both UK and European Union law.

Seafarers

Work at sea involves not only some duties that are safety-critical but also periods remote from onshore healthcare and travel to parts of the world with differing climates and patterns of infection. Food preparation is normally carried out on board. Medical fitness is assessed every two years by doctors approved by the Maritime and Coastguard Agency (MCA). National medical standards form the basis for this assessment.[3] These are concerned with recurrence risks, which could increase the probability of illness while at sea, as well as with forms of impairment that could interfere with duties such as navigation, engineering, food preparation and responding to emergencies. National standards are in accord with international requirements of the International Labour Office and the International Maritime Organization.

Commercial yachtmasters, crew on coastal and inland passenger vessels and on inshore workboats provide the office issuing their certificates of competency with a form completed by a doctor, normally their general practitioner, to show whether they have any health problems. The office forwards this to a medical assessor appointed by the MCA for a decision if any relevant health problems are identified. Apart from sight tests for masters and mates, there are no medical fitness standards for UK fishermen at present.

Offshore workers

Agreed medical standards for working on offshore structures, normally oil and gas exploration or production platforms, have been developed by the employers' organization, the United Kingdom Offshore Operators Association (UKOOA).[4] These are particularly concerned with risks of recurrent illness when working offshore as well as with the fitness requirements of rescue and fire-fighting teams. A network of doctors is maintained by UKOOA to undertake these medicals.

Divers

The extreme working environment for commercial divers means that there are fitness requirements to undertake work under water, using unusual gas mixtures when the diving is deep. They may also live as well as work, if diving is very deep, under saturation conditions to avoid decompression. Here divers live under raised pressure, breathing a diving gas mixture for several days, and it is important to avoid the risk of any recurrent illnesses, as prolonged decompression would be needed before they could receive medical care, unless the medical team is also compressed.[5] The Health and Safety Executive (HSE) is responsible for approving doctors to perform the annual medical examinations required for commercial divers. These medicals aim to check that a diver's health has not been damaged by their work, as well as to assess their fitness.

Physically demanding public safety work

Emergency service personnel (police, fire, ambulance, coastguard) are assessed not only for their fitness to drive but also for their fitness to carry out their other duties, especially those where physical limitations or poor decision-taking can put other people at risk. Similar considerations apply to the armed forces and to other workers, such as security staff who may have safety or enforcement responsibilities.

Control room work

Poor decision-taking in control rooms of chemical and power plants and in those coordinating transport (eg air traffic controllers, rail signallers, both of whom are covered by the medical criteria for their sectors of transport) or emergency services can put the public at increased risk, just as can similar weaknesses with transport control at sea, in the air, and on the road and rail networks. Observed training and simulation exercises play a big part in assessing suitability, but it is usual also to have medical assessments to pick up any sensory, cognitive or behavioural problems which could impair sound decisions being taken.

References

1. Cox RAF, Edwards FC, Palmer K, eds. *Fitness for Work: The Medical Aspects*. Oxford: Oxford University Press, 2000.

2. Railway Group Standards. Rail Safety and Standards Board. GO/RT 3251 – Drivers, GE/RT 8067 Personal Track Safety, GE/RT 8070 Drugs and Alcohol. www.rgsonline.co.uk/

3. *Seafarer Medical Examination System and Medical and Eyesight Standards*. MSN 1765. Maritime and Coastguard Agency, 2002. www.mcga.gov.uk/c4mca/mcga-seafarer_information/mcga-dqs_st_shs_seafarer_information-medical.htm

4. *Guidelines for Medical Aspects of Fitness for Offshore Work*, Issue No. 5. United Kingdom Offshore Operators Association, 2003.

5. *The Medical Examination and Assessment of Divers (MA1)*. Health and Safety Executive, 2005. www.hse.gov.uk/diving/ma1.pdf

Index